Loving an Addict, Loving Yourself

The Top 10 Survival Tips for Loving Someone with an Addiction

"Money is inextricably linked to every aspect of a person's life. As financial planners, we have the privilege of getting to know our clients at a very personal level. It is amazing how many people encounter addiction either in their workplace or in their families. We keep Candace's book in our front lobby and in our lending library. These copies regularly disappear. And I know why. Candace Plattor has a gift for summarizing difficult, sometimes complex truths in an easy to read, palatable format. You can tell she knows what she is talking about and has the experience to back it. If you or a family member is curious about whether addiction is an issue, I would highly recommend picking up this book. Just don't ask us for it, because it has probably gone missing!"

~ TRACY THEEMES, MA, CFP, FMA, FCSI
Financial Advisor, Sophia Financial Group,
Raymond James Ltd, www.sophiafinancial.ca

"Hi Candace, I want to tell you how much I've enjoyed your book—I think I should buy a case of them to hand out to all of our family! I have been at two family workshops, where I have learned a lot as well, and my daughter has been to treatment for substance abuse. It has been quite a journey to come to understand what my job is now as a mother. I just felt so compelled to email you and tell you that you wrote an awesome book—and I will continue to share what I'm learning from it with others... thanks again!"

~ GM

"Candace's ability to name the presence of addictive behaviours—regardless of who the addicts are in relationship with—was tremendously significant and freeing for me, both on a personal level and in my professional life as a therapist. She identifies clearly who is responsible for what, from the perspective of both the addict and the family member, and takes away the crippling effects of blame. Her book has helped me tremendously and I recommend it highly to my clients."

~ HEATHER DICKSON, MA
Therapist in Private Practice

"*Loving an Addict, Loving Yourself* is such a straightforward approach to dealing with an addiction situation with a loved one or ourselves. One of Candace's favorite sayings in the book is that "If nothing changes, nothing changes". The book is about our desire to change our lives from where we have drifted into the paralysis of addictive and/or codependent behaviors, to be able to take active steps of self-realization and self-care. Candace gives us the 10 most important survival tips on 'how to' get from here to there in this easy to read guide. Reading it was an epiphany for me—I understand now that one can choose to change from 'drift' to 'direction' and survive as a stronger and more loving person. I give away new copies to friends and family because my book stays by my bedside to be read and reread."

~ KATHRYN FRIESEN, MSc

"*Candace Plattor's work has effected a powerful positive change in my life. **Loving An Addict, Loving Yourself** was my crucial first step in breaking free from the pain of an addictive relationship. This little blue book is so wise and wonderful. It was instrumental in creating the joyful life I'm now living. Thank you Candace!*"

~ Alexandra

"*I just finished reading the two forewords and your acknowledgement in your book and I was deeply moved by all that I read. In fact it even brought tears to my eyes. Inspirational tears...*

I'm so grateful to have you as my therapist at this stage in my life. For without you, I can't even begin to imagine what my life would be like because you have taught me so much about myself and helped me to start growing up. And I have grown in ways I've yearned to grow, and I couldn't have done it without you. Thank you for your book, what a treasure it is!"

~ KT

"*I want you to know that I have read your book and find it really well-organized, practical and easy to understand for the lay person... from what I have read so far, you have made an outstanding contribution to the world of helping with addictions.*"

~ DC

"*I wanted to let you know how much I have enjoyed your book. I will definitely buy another copy to lend to others (or better still, to show them and then have them make a note to buy their own). My signed copy will be staying on my shelf.*

I found it very easy to read and a sensible approach for so many of us stuck in our "trying to fix or support" role. I believe when someone is caught in the enabling role of a loved one, they can be helped by a sensible, clear approach. I like yours.

I also like your quotes. And personal stories...."

~ KARLEEN NEVERY, RPC CGA,
Therapist in Private Practice

"I read your book **Loving an Addict, Loving Yourself: The Top 10 Survival Tips for Loving Someone with an Addiction** from start to finish the very first night I got it. I couldn't put it down because I kept wanting to know about the next survival tip! It was a very positive read and it left me feeling relieved. I still read part of your book each night to keep my spirit uplifted. I especially like the case studies because they give me a sense of how to go about working on my relationship in a healthy way, rather than continuing the patterns I got used to. I especially like how each case study ends off with a positive outcome for the loved one of the addicted person. Thank you for your help."

~ MC

"As I read this book, I gradually became convinced that the key to my well-being was Self-Care. I am happy to say that as I started to recognize and take care of my own needs, life with the addict I love improved. But even if it hadn't, I would have been happier, healthier, and more at peace. Candace is a champion for this process, and she is living proof that it works.

~ SK

I love this book; it's smart, it's current and relevant, and it's chock-full of practical information. Candace's wisdom and experience shine through. I often read passages out to my groups and I recommend it to loved ones of those struggling with addiction. It definitely filled a gap in reference material in this field."

~ FIONA JEYACHANDRAN, ALCOHOL & DRUG COUNSELLOR

Loving an Addict,

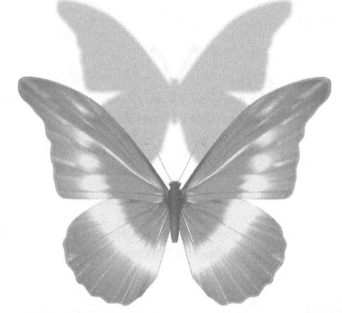

Loving Yourself

The Top 10 Survival Tips
for Loving Someone with an Addiction

Revised Edition

Candace Plattor, M.A.

Library and Archives Canada Cataloguing in Publication

Plattor, Candace, 1950-, author
      Loving an addict, loving yourself : the top 10 survival tips for loving someone with an addiction / Candace Plattor. -- Revised edition.

Originally published in 2010.

ISBN 978-0-9813850-6-8 (pbk.)

      1. Addicts--Family relationships. 2. Substance abuse--Patients--Family relationships. 3. Self-help techniques. 4. Self-care, Health.
5. Interpersonal confrontation. I. Title.

RC533.P532 2014   362.29'13   C2014-908119-7

Published by:
Candace Plattor, M.A.
604-677-5876
candace@candaceplattor.com
www.candaceplattor.com

Editing by Arlene Prunkl; Cover and content design by Bobbie Cann

Dedication

I dedicate this book to my dear sisters José and Melanie. You tirelessly read and re-read my manuscript as I wrote it, line by line, chapter by chapter, giving me incredibly useful feedback, suggestions, and loving encouragement. I could not have done this without your help, and I certainly would not have had as much fun without you.

If nothing ever
changed
there would be no
butterflies

~anonymous

Contents

Foreword

FOREWORD BY CAROLINE SUTHERLAND

Addiction is something with which I have had no personal experience in my adult life. I have not been an alcoholic, a drug addict, or
an over-spender, but in my youth I was an over-eater. I would go on
stringent diets to lose a few pounds, but at the end of the week because I had starved myself for days, I would eat a whole pie!

My heart goes out to anyone who has a major addiction. And to those
who have had the courage to set an addiction aside I say, "Bravo!"

An addiction is something that has a hold over us, something that is
difficult to set aside, and something that we are powerless to stop—
unless we are given some tools and encouragement. As a nutritional
counselor and health educator, I see plenty of people with food addictions—mainly to sugar as their drug of choice.

The addiction to sugar on a higher level really represents sweetness
in life. If we can find the truly wonderful things that life has to offer

and immerse ourselves in these pursuits, we will be brimming with happiness and there will be no need for the excessive sugar in desserts, candy, alcohol, and other sweets.

Life is all "done with mirrors." What we crave on the inside we fill ourselves with on the outside.

Addictions are very powerful, and they take us off the track we really belong on. But having the courage to face an addiction, to stare it down, and to overcome it, can lead us to liberation and bring us to our higher purpose.

Candace Plattor, author of *Loving an Addict, Loving Yourself: The Top 10 Survival Tips for Loving Someone with an Addiction,* has done just that.

I first met Candace through one of my clients over a year ago. We arranged a meeting to discuss ways to improve Candace's health and her energy. Even though for years she had been a great advocate for health and nutrition, I was instantly captivated by Candace's enthusiasm and her dedication to following my suggestions. As a result, her health has improved immensely and she has learned a completely new way of understanding her body and its needs.

In order to overcome an addiction and have the clarity we need to make positive life choices and evaluate situations that could be potentially harmful for us, we need a strong, healthy body and a clear mind. Candace's work with EMDR and other unique counseling tools that she uses, along with her amazing dedication to her own holistic self-care, offer an important and distinctive way out of the maze of addictive behaviors and onto the new path ahead.

Caroline Sutherland

Author, The Body Knows and *The Body Knows…How to Stay Young*

Foreword by Suzanne Jean

I am honored to have been asked to endorse Candace Plattor's book, *Loving an Addict, Loving Yourself.*

Over the past sixteen years, I have witnessed amazing transformations in Candace both personally and professionally. For much of that time we worked together at Watari Research Association, an agency in the low-income Downtown Eastside area of Vancouver, Canada, whose mission is to facilitate positive change in the lives of at-risk children, youth, and families through innovative counseling and programs.

Candace and I initially connected through debriefing our difficult work together. We quickly realized that we share a deep belief in an individual's innate strength, resilience, capabilities, and desire for wellness, no matter what the circumstances are. I have never seen Candace back down from a client-related problem, regardless of how complex it might be, when serving people who are living with challenges such as addiction and abuse. If she does not understand something, she will seek out the required expertise or develop the skill herself to do whatever is needed to truly help the individual or family. This tenacious quality of Candace's, as well as a genuine commitment to lifelong learning, contribute much to her wonderful discoveries in the field of addictions.

I would characterize Candace's professional approach as similar to a secret formula: Just the right measure and combination of compassion, reality, and humor delivered at just the right moment. Whether she is working with the addict or the addict's loved ones, I believe Candace has achieved success and credibility as a counselor because of her ability to deeply access both her intuition and her personal experience with addiction and recovery, allowing her to connect with others—without judgment—at a profound human level. She relates from a place of strong consistent values that provide her clients with a sense of comfort and safety.

This book represents Candace's integrity as an addictions therapist by incorporating the positive values she upholds. As well, *Loving an Addict, Loving Yourself* offers an honest, practical guide for those who may be feeling the hopelessness and isolation that occur from loving someone with an addiction. Knowing that Candace values being able to share her knowledge and wisdom in order to be of service to others, I have no doubt that the information in this book will be tremendously useful to the loved ones of people with any type of addictive behaviors.

Suzanne Jean

Former Executive Director, Watari Research Association

CEO, Kaizen Holdings

Acknowledgments

Writing my first book *Loving an Addict, Loving Yourself* has been a profoundly transformative experience for me on both a personal and professional level. The process, as well as the finished product, serves as a culmination of my many years of working with addicts and their loved ones, as well as my 22+ years of doing my own personal recovery work. Just like all other addicts who want a better life, it became imperative for me to discover the underlying reasons for why I needed to use addictive behaviors in the first place, in order to be able to stop engaging in them. My sincere hope is always that my journey of recovery from addiction can help someone else, just as other peoples' journeys have inspired me. I have no doubt that the best is yet to come!

There are many people who helped and supported me on this particular leg of my journey, and I treasure the richness you have all brought to my life.

First and foremost, I would like to thank both my mother, Emma, and Bill for believing in me and encouraging me every step of the way. I appreciate your willingness to read and edit parts of this manuscript. Your support means more to me than I can say.

My father, Stan, led the way for me to become a therapist by role-modelling what that life was like for him. I love you and I miss you every day.

I would have been lost without my brilliant and creative business coach, Juliet Austin, who has been at my side for the past several years, guiding me in my professional journey. My deep thanks to you for helping me so much whenever I needed you.

To my dear friends Ingrid, Jodi, and CJ – my heartfelt thanks to you for being with me on my path for many years. You have each taught me much about life, love, compassion, and friendship, and I am a far better person for knowing you.

I am deeply indebted to Caroline Sutherland, whose ever-generous assistance and support have helped me to restore my physical body to a wonderful level of health I have not known since I was first diagnosed with Crohn's Disease in 1973. You have given me my life back. I am so very grateful to have benefitted from your intuitive gifts and your clarity. There will never be enough words to thank you.

How fortunate I have been to know Bree Willson for the past several months. It's wonderful to be able to benefit from your vast wisdom and your gentleness of spirit, and I am grateful that you are in my life.

The very helpful insights and suggestions from my wonderful "book-team" of Arlene (my talented editor), Bobbie (my imaginative designer), and Carole (my resourceful Virtual Assistant) have made my life much easier – thank you all!

My heartfelt gratitude goes to Dr. Stan Lubin, who became my personal physician in the very early days of my recovery from addiction. You have seen me at my best, at my worst, and everywhere in between, and you have always believed in me. I deeply appreciate the gentleness, compassion, and respect you give to me every time I see you, and I thank you so much for all your help throughout the years.

I am indebted to Suzanne, Lawrence, Lauren, Michelle, and all the caring and dedicated staff at Watari. With your help and support, I was given the opportunity to hone my skills as an Addictions Counselor and to learn many important personal lessons. Please keep up the wonderful work you're doing.

Kudos to Dr. Jenny Melamed, for being an incomparably ethical Addictions Doctor with a heart of gold. Your patients love you and I understand why. I feel privileged to be working beside you.

I warmly acknowledge the brilliant assistance I receive from Dr. Bob Armstrong. Your amazing wisdom, clarity, and delightful sense of humour are of great value to me as your client. In my darkest moments, you are somehow able to take the jumbled mess of my emotional growth periods and turn them into something that makes sense. You have an incredible gift and I am in awe of your skill as a therapist/clinical supervisor.

I have saved my most profound appreciation till the end: My deepest thanks and admiration go to all of my extremely courageous clients, both past and present, for trusting and believing in me and in yourselves. Without exception, you have each taught me so much over the years as our journeys have intertwined. As much as I love doing the work I do, there is a bittersweet part of being a therapist: As people do their brave and daring inner work, they become stronger and more capable of living their best lives—and that is precisely when they are able to move on without me. I fully recognize that this is exactly the way it is supposed to be, and sometimes it is hard to say goodbye. But I keep you all in my heart and am always grateful for the time we've spent together. Thank you for sharing yourselves with me.

Please be happy and healthy, Everyone!

2015 Acknowledgements:

In addition to those mentioned above, five years later in 2015 there are now a few more people I'd like to acknowledge:

My wonderful support system which includes: CJ, Ina, Jodi, Jose, Mika, Glo, Alyson, Tierney, Pamela, and Cait. I am truly blessed.

To Bobby, Shamira, and Kimen—my deep thanks for keeping me as healthy as this body can be. You never give up on me, even when my situation is difficult.

Katharyn, I appreciate your assistance with the fulfillment of this book: the receiving and the shipping. It's wonderful to know that you'll pick up those essential responsibilities.

Ingrid, thanks for signing on to design this revised edition—great job!

To Steve Harrison and all of the wonderful Quantum Leap coaches: Geoffrey, Danette, Raia, Brian, Mary, and Martha—you are all amazing teachers and I'm grateful for your guidance.

And two big extra helpings of gratitude go to my virtual assistant, Carole, and to my social media expert, Tracey—both of you make my sometimes crazy-busy life much less chaotic. I'm happy I can rely on you both—you are true gifts in my life!

My Story

Have you ever reached such a low point in your life that you weren't sure you could rise up from it? If so, I can definitely relate. In fact, I am a perfect example of that age-old saying: "What doesn't kill us makes us stronger!"

I grew up in a family with many of the same kinds of dysfunctional patterns that most other families had back in the fifties and sixties—some of which still persist today.

Although my parents were both educators, entrenched in academia, there was addiction in my family. My mother was an inarguable workaholic and used addictive medications like Valium on a consistent basis, while my father enjoyed both gambling and involving himself in numerous extramarital affairs. My parents didn't like each other very much, and what I believe today is that they mutually decided to use these behaviors to keep each other at arm's length. What they didn't seem to understand—or care much about—was that this also kept them both from being present for my brother and me. That sense of dysfunctional distance in our family—as well as the emotional and verbal abuse that frequently accompanied the sometimes-brutal isolation—created scars for us kids that we unwittingly carried well into adulthood.

For some reason unknown to me, we moved around a lot as a family—from Brooklyn, NY where I was born, to Alabama to New Orleans, and many places in between. We never stayed longer than two years in any one place and, in fact, there was one place we stayed in for six weeks—and that was after we'd unpacked and settled in because we thought we'd be there for a while! All of this upheaval meant that I was constantly the new kid on the block, which was quite stressful for the shy little girl I was, especially with self-absorbed parents who didn't seem to care how I was faring. I always felt like a stranger in a strange land, like I just didn't fit in anywhere. This created a lot of social anxiety for me and has been one of the deepest scars for me to heal. But as difficult as my childhood was, it wasn't until my early twenties that I discovered what stress truly was—when life as I'd known it came crashing down around me.

A few years before that happened, my parents finally decided to separate and to ultimately divorce. I recently heard Dr. Phil say that children would rather come from a broken home than live in one. I concur. After living in a broken home for so long, this separation felt like a relief to me. Although it was also fraught with sadness, confusion, and fear, it was a reprieve in some ways.

My mother wanted to get as far away from my father as she could, and since I was not quite eighteen and therefore legally under the age of consent, I had no choice but to go with her. Dad was still living in New Orleans, so my mother, brother, and I crossed virtually the entire continent of North America and came to Canada, where my mother procured a job as a professor at the University of Calgary.

I had recently graduated from high school in New Orleans and was ready for my own university experience, so I decided to attend the University of Calgary. As a drama student in the Bachelor of Fine Arts program, I was in heaven. I made new friends and had a wonderful extensive social life living in residence, attending classes, and performing in a variety of theatrical productions. I was happy and finally felt like I belonged somewhere—a first for me.

Unfortunately, this happiness was short-lived. After graduating from university in 1973, I became engaged to a man who was on a visa from the US and couldn't stay in Canada. We decided to travel from Alberta, in western Canada, to the east coast of the US where his family lived. Once again, I was going to be crisscrossing the continent, moving to yet another new place.

How excited I was at first, looking forward to spending exclusive time with him before meeting my new soon-to-be family! I had such hopes of belonging, of being part of his family as his wife. What I didn't understand at the time was that, like so many others of us from dysfunctional homes, I'd chosen a partner who had some of the worst characteristics of both of my parents. This man I'd chosen to marry was emotionally and verbally abusive with me, shaming me frequently with snide remarks. But, because I'd grown up with exactly that, I unwittingly found myself deep within my comfort zone. At that time, I actually thought his nastiness meant that he loved me—yet another childhood scar I'd need to heal.

So there we were, embarking on our long and winding road trip, with everything we owned packed into a VW van. The trip was fine for a while—as fine as things can be in an abusive relationship. But toward the middle of our journey, with no warning whatsoever, I suddenly became violently ill—which made things exceedingly difficult—and I didn't get any better as time went on. Just imagine riding in an old, rickety, beat-up VW van for days on end, feeling like you were suffering with unrelenting symptoms of severe food poisoning. That was my reality for the remainder of this cross-country trip. I was miserable, and my fiancé didn't seem to care much. In fact, most of the time I felt like a burden to him—just like I'd felt with my busy, self-centered parents.

Many of us seem destined to repeat these old family-of-origin dynamics until we ultimately heal them. For me, that particular healing took quite a while.

When we finally reached our destination, I was so sick that I simply had no energy left to make nice with my future in-laws—who, it turned out, were not the most compassionate people. They wanted me to be a certain way for their prized son—but I just couldn't please them in the condition I was in. I felt like a dismal failure in every possible way, and it didn't take long for my fiancé to tell me he wanted a healthy woman, not one like me.

Not surprisingly, we broke up and I came back home to Canada absolutely devastated. After many months of chronic, unrelenting illness and a multitude of doctor appointments, I was finally diagnosed with Crohn's Disease—a "new kid on the block" condition that doctors had no clue how to treat.

I'm sure it must have been difficult for those doctors to have a young woman like myself coming to see them, often in tears, complaining of terrible pain, depressed, feeling like her life was passing her by— and not know what to do to help her. They must have felt like they needed to do *something, anything.*

So what they did was give me plenty of medications that turned out to be highly addictive. In their defense, addiction wasn't on the radar back then like it is today; they probably didn't have any idea at that point of the toll this would have on me. But even forty years ago those meds caused me no end of serious problems that would take me a lot of years to unravel.

Being the good girl I was back then, I faithfully took all of the Valium, Codeine, and Demerol (a strong painkiller, perhaps equivalent to today's Oxycontin) they endlessly prescribed for me—day after day, month after month, year after year.

Fast forward about fifteen years—I was still sick, deeply addicted to pills and also to marijuana, which I'd initially discovered during my university days, and which took away a lot of the pain and shame associated with an illness like Crohn's. Although I can definitely understand and relate to the concept of medical marijuana, I know beyond question that pot is addictive—and the pot that's around today is even stronger and more addictive than what I was smoking forty years ago. As well, I was extremely depressed, which made sense since all of those substances act as depressants in the system. Anybody's body would have been adversely affected by this combination of drugs. And to top all of that off, nothing was getting any better in my life—and it felt to me like things would just continue that way forever.

Then came an experience that frightened me deeply. I was taking a break at work one day, not feeling well physically and pretty drained emotionally—par for the course for me in those days—and I found myself seriously thinking about suicide for the first time. I was lying down on a couch in the staff room with my eyes closed, trying to rest so I could get through my shift, when it suddenly occurred to me that I had enough pills to do the job—and if I timed it right, no one would find me in time and I'd be dead.

That day, I thought I might actually do it.

And that scared me.

But somewhere deep inside of me, I knew I had an extremely important choice to make, right then and there. And I'm so grateful that I made the right one.

I left work early, came directly home and immediately called the Vancouver Crisis Line, sobbing, struggling to describe what was really going on with me. The person I talked with that day literally saved my life by strongly suggesting I go to SAFER, a suicide prevention counseling center here in Vancouver, which I chose to do the next day. I was so relieved that there might actually be some help for me! From there I was guided to voluntarily sign myself into the psychiatric ward of a local hospital, where I stayed for nearly four weeks, receiving medical attention for my Crohn's and much-needed counseling. It was there that I first learned about addiction, as I began to understand that I had indeed become a drug addict. I also met a couple of other patients who were trying to kick their own substance addictions. They were going to Narcotics Anonymous meetings every day at noon, right across the street—so I decided to join them.

That was really the beginning of my recovery from addiction. As I sat in those meetings, day after day, depressed, crying, sharing my pain as best I could, the others would remind me to *keep coming back*. They would say wise things like, "Don't give up five minutes before the miracle happens," and "Just for today, my needs are met." Tattooed bikers in black leather and heavy chains would hug me after meetings, offering me the kind of compassionate response I had not received in my own family. It was amazing and very healing. Although being "part of" was something I'd always had difficulty with, I found myself feeling a certain sense of belonging for the first time since my university days.

Three years into my recovery, I began to give back to my community by working as an addictions counselor in Vancouver's poverty-stricken Downtown Eastside. This area of Vancouver is known as the lowest income postal code in Canada with the highest number, per capita, of addicts, alcoholics, and homeless people. I worked there for sixteen years getting the kind of education about addiction

I could never have received anywhere else—for which I continue to be grateful.

As I had been several years before, my clients in the Downtown Eastside were addicts and alcoholics who were still entrenched in active addiction. I found that some of them really wanted help getting off that horrible treadmill, while others were not as interested in stopping. The latter group of clients basically wanted to tell me their, "Can you *believe* this?" stories week after week, presenting themselves as victims of what had happened to them. Often, the clients who made the choice to take counseling seriously and stop using and drinking had experienced severe hardships as well, but instead chose to empower themselves rather than see themselves as prisoners of their past circumstances. I found that distinction both fascinating and significant, and it would definitely influence my later work in the addictions field.

My work also helped to keep me clean and sober, to choose to stay on the path of recovery.

As time went on, the families of my addicted clients also began to call me, wanting to set up sessions with me to discuss what was happening with their addicts. This was a bit strange for me at first because I too was the loved one of addicts, and I really wasn't at all sure what to do for them. But as those sessions progressed, I started to see some striking patterns going on in virtually all of those relationships. The loved ones were almost always enabling the addicts by doing things like making excuses for their difficult behavior, giving them money on a regular basis, or allowing them to live rent-free in the family home with no expectations of them contributing anything financially or otherwise, even putting up with their verbally and physically abusive ways. I instinctively understood that this was not helping the situation to change in any way. I began to wonder, "If I had been enabled like that in my own addiction, would I have chosen to stop?" The clear answer was, "Not on your life!"

I knew I was on to something vitally important.

After working for twenty-five years with people who have addicts in their lives, this is what I know to be true: When people who love addicts enable them, as I had unintentionally done with my own addicted loved ones, it keeps the addiction going rather than help it to stop.

Family and friends enable because they are frightened and desperate—and because they simply don't know what else to do. But somewhere deep inside they know that what they're doing with the addicts they love so dearly may actually be hurting them. During their first session with me they often say, "I know I'm enabling but…" and then give me all of their rationales and explanations for why they're doing that. When my clients do this, I set them straight as soon as I can—because addiction (especially to mind-altering substances) is often a life-or-death situation. I personally don't believe we have the luxury of waiting to shift both our perspective and our behaviors into those that will truly assist the addiction to stop.

There is still, at the time of this writing, very little help for you, the loved one of an addict. There is a lot of help out there for those who are addicted: detoxes, treatment centers, counseling, self-help support groups. But, relatively speaking, there are few resources for their loved ones, who are also struggling and feeling lost. It didn't take me long to know that I needed to do what I could to remedy this situation.

When I fully understood that *enabling is never a loving act* toward an addict, I decided to write a book for the loved ones of people with addictions, outlining how they themselves could change the ways they were contributing to their circumstances so that both they and the addicts they cared about could get well. I published the original version of *Loving an Addict, Loving Yourself: The Top 10 Survival Tips for Loving Someone with an Addiction* in January of 2010, and when the family members I counseled told me how helpful this book was to them, I wrote and published the accompanying volume *Loving an Addict, Loving Yourself: The Workbook* a couple of years later.

To my surprise, both of my books have won International and USA Book Awards, and are now being used in a variety of treatment centers throughout the world as part of their family programs.

When I was in my own active addiction—and even in the first few years of my early recovery—if anyone had told me that I would actually do something important to help the world, I would have thought they were crazy!

Me? Hopeless, depressed, suicidal, addicted ME??

But here I am. I'm living proof that remaining in addiction or shifting into recovery is, ultimately, nothing more than a choice.

I don't believe that addicts choose to become addicted. I certainly didn't. But once addicts find themselves there, they are deciding at each moment whether to stay in active addiction or go into some kind of active recovery. I chose recovery many years ago; today, one day at a time, I am twenty-seven years clean and sober.

I'm here to tell you that people can change—addicts *can* change. Please don't give up hope just yet—don't leave five minutes before the miracle happens.

Welcome to Your Life— A Dramatically Fresh Approach to Loving an Addicted Person

Writing this book has been a dream of mine for a long time. As a recovering addict myself with over twenty years of freedom from drugs, alcohol, and many other addictive behaviors, I remember very well how it feels not to like either myself or my life. I know the difference between having healthy relationships with my loved ones as opposed to tolerating, and even contributing to, difficult and dysfunctional relationships. Today I understand that if I want my life to be different, I must be the change I want to see. Today I know that everything in my life begins with me—and that self-trust must be earned, just as trust from another person is also earned.

SELF-RESPECT—WHAT A CONCEPT!

I have experienced the immense difference between living with self-respect and living without it. For me there is no question at all—having my self-respect is far better. And now that I fully have my self-respect, it is non-negotiable in all of my relationships, especially in the relationship I have with myself. And I know, without a doubt, that no one can take my self-respect away from me without my permission.

In addition to having had my own personal struggles with addictive behaviors, I have also been involved in close, intimate relationships with others who have had problems with addiction. When we love an addict, without inner work our self-respect is at best fleeting. For some people, it will be virtually nonexistent even when life seems to be going really well for them. In my experience, the vast majority of people never even think about it, much less realize how vitally important it is to fully own our self-respect. And when we love an addict, so much of our energy and effort goes into trying to change them that we often don't pay much attention to ourselves. Our own needs, desires, yearnings, and yes, our self-respect, generally wind up on the back burner.

WHAT I'VE LEARNED ABOUT ADDICTS AND THEIR LOVED ONES

The Downtown Eastside area of Vancouver[1] is statistically the lowest-income region in all of Canada. It has the largest number of people on income assistance, the highest percentage of the "working poor," and the highest concentration of practicing alcoholics and drug addicts in the country.

While working as an addictions counselor in Vancouver's gritty Downtown Eastside for more than fifteen years, I had many opportunities to meet not only clients who were struggling with their own addictions, but also the families, partners, and friends of those addicts. I soon understood that addiction has many far-reaching ripple effects for all concerned. Loving an addict means sharing in the misery of the addiction, until our own healing allows for a different way of life.

Coupling my personal knowledge of what it's like to love someone who has an addictive behavior with my professional understanding gleaned from working with families of addicts, what I know for certain is that we, their loved ones, are strong and capable people. We have to be. We are able to withstand unspeakable misery and grief.

---

1   The Downtown Eastside is Vancouver, British Columbia's oldest neighbourhood. It is known for its high incidences of poverty, drug use, sex trade, HIV infection, crime, as well as a history of community activism.
     Source: http://en.wikipedia.org/wiki/Downtown_Eastside. 09/23/09

We are determined to try anything we can to make our situations better, and sometimes we can be quite creative in the ways we do that.

As I continue to work with addicts and their families in my practice today, I find that it is necessary for me to teach loved ones how to distinguish between their own *helping* behaviors and what they may be doing to *enable* the addicts in their lives to actually continue their addictions. Until that work is done, the families and loved ones are unable to attain the outcomes they truly want. The inner work for them generally involves changing some of their own entrenched and dysfunctional patterns so they can deal more effectively with their addicted loved ones.

Later we will look more closely at what kinds of behaviors constitute *enabling*, and how to shift these into healthier strategies that will allow both you and the addicted person in your life to achieve a happier and more harmonious relationship.

You Can Only Change Yourself

Contrary to the thinking of many people who love an addict, *you are really the only person you can change.* Trying to change someone else is a complete waste of time. Like most people who love an addict, you have probably become skilled at trying to change the other person, but the question is, has it truly worked for you yet? No? I didn't think so. It isn't because you haven't tried hard enough; it's because it is simply impossible to change other people if they are not ready to change.

The true shift in your relationships will come only with *the courage to look at yourself honestly and realistically,* to see how you may have been contributing to the problem. By choosing to do this difficult but rewarding work, you will be able to create solutions that are more effective.

Since you are reading this book, perhaps you have questioned your relationship with your addicted loved one and wondered if your time could be better spent focusing on yourself and increasing your own self-respect. If you are like most people, your answer will be a resounding "Yes!" followed quickly by "But *how* do I do that?"

AN INVITATION

By taking the journey with me into *Loving an Addict, Loving Yourself: The Top 10 Survival Tips for Loving Someone with an Addiction*, you will learn how to do exactly that—focus on yourself and increase your self-respect.

In writing *Loving an Addict, Loving Yourself*, I offer you an invitation to reclaim those long-forgotten needs, desires, and yearnings. This is an invitation to live the life you want to live by focusing more on yourself than on the addict in your life. You do not have to remain addicted to someone else's addiction.

I invite you to begin living your life in a dramatically new, more self-respecting way. Are you ready? Let's get started!

CHAPTER 1

Loving Someone with an Addiction: A Life of Chaos

L et's face it—life with an addict is hard. No matter what the outward addiction is, the underlying dynamic of an addict's life is one of chaos. Addicts who continue to be involved with their own destructive behaviors typically experience many emotional highs and lows, creating a virtual rollercoaster of "pink clouds" followed by severe despondency, remorse, and self-loathing, with every conceivable emotion in between. Unfortunately, if you love an addict, you are likely to experience these highs and lows as well.

For example, many people with addictive behaviors develop health issues over time for a variety of reasons. These could be the result of either the physical strain of eating disorders such as anorexia or bulimia, the misuse of toxic substances such as alcohol, drugs, or cigarettes; or the enduring stress they experience from feeling the shame of engaging in such dysfunctional activities as compulsive over-spending, gambling, or Internet addiction.

In many cases, financial difficulties also arise, which can have far-reaching implications. When addicts feed their addiction, they may forget to feed their families. They may also overlook important financial concerns such as paying the rent or the mortgage. Budgets fly out the window, over-spending often becomes the norm, and monetary mayhem ensues. For someone who cares for an addict, this chaos can feel as though it is ruining your life.

The Dynamics of Addiction

The Beginning Stages: The Start of Denial

In the beginning stages of addiction, addicts tend to dabble in their dysfunctional behaviors without being aware or concerned about the implications of potential addiction. Here are some typical examples:

> Greg starts his drug use by doing only a few lines of his friend's cocaine occasionally at parties. "Nothing to worry about," he assures himself and anyone else who dares to comment about it. Each time he indulges in cocaine, he likes it even more.

> Janet's over-spending starts with a number of small shopping sprees that gradually begin to take the shape of more and more bags of items just sitting, unpacked, in the corner of her bedroom. She somehow feels more secure just having them there and tells herself she will get around to organizing them soon. Meanwhile, the shopping continues.

> Don's gambling begins innocently as weekly poker nights with his buddies. He greatly enjoys the camaraderie and loves the feeling of winning, but he is becoming increasingly aware that he does not at all enjoy losing money.

> At the initial stages of her eating disorder, Lisa is happy to discover that she can eat what she wants without having to be concerned about gaining weight. She feels pleased that she has found a foolproof way to keep her overeating under control; all she has to do is throw up after each meal, which seems like a fair exchange.

The Progressive Stages: The Addiction Worsens
The nature of addiction is that it is *progressive*. This means that the symptoms worsen as the addictive behaviors are pursued with increasing frequency.

> As time goes on, Greg has progressed from being a social cocaine user; he now indulges every weekend, and sometimes during the week as well. Even though he is starting to feel a little concerned about it, he would never admit that to anyone.

> Janet's shopping becomes increasingly problematic as new shoes, clothing, and accessories continue to fill up much of her closet space. Four $1,000 outfits are now hanging there, unworn, with their tags still attached.

> Don has graduated from weekly poker nights to full weekends spent at the local casino. He is aware that his losses far outweigh his wins as he tries to hide his dwindling cash reserves, as well as his absences from home, from his wife. Yet he is compelled to continue, telling himself that next time he might win.

> Lisa now binges several times a week and always looks forward to the time when she can purge because the overeating has become worse: food has become her best friend, providing the comfort she craves in her life. Although she is finding that throwing up this often causes a burning sensation in her throat and in her stomach, she attempts to convince herself that being able to eat what she wants without gaining weight is still the way to go. The fact that she has recently gone down a couple of dress sizes encourages her to continue her addictive behavior.

The Advanced Stages: Consequences Abound

By now, Greg has increased his cocaine intake substantially. He doesn't wait for parties anymore; instead, his daily usage has increased and he has learned to hide it from his family, friends, and colleagues at work. He sometimes wonders if any of his drug buddies use as much cocaine as he does, but doesn't ask anyone for fear of being discovered. Because he is rarely hungry when he is high on coke, he has undergone a noticeable weight loss. His metabolism has also been damaged by the amount of the drug he keeps putting in his system. He feels nervous and anxious much of the time, and his family is noticing that he is much more short-tempered than he used to be. Greg is beginning to worry that other people know about his "secret" cocaine use.

Janet has now maxed out all of her major credit cards. She often finds herself awake at 3 a.m., worrying that her husband will find out. Although she is still functioning well at work, an obsessive fear of losing her job occupies many of her waking thoughts; without an income, Janet knows she will not be able to pay off her credit cards or continue her beloved buying excursions. She understands that she needs to stop spending but can't imagine her life without shopping. She has no idea whom she can talk to about this or where she can turn for help, so she keeps all of her fears to herself. And she continues to shop.

Don can't seem to stop gambling. He is totally consumed with thoughts of his next trip to the casino. He obsessively goes over and over mistakes he feels he made at the tables the last time he was there, and lives with the constant compulsion to return as soon as possible. He knows he will do whatever it takes to continue his consistent gambling, even if it means lying to his family and losing money that isn't really his to wager in the first place. He is becoming aware that he is on a downward spiral that could cost him everything.

Lisa's troubles are at an all-time high: she is now bingeing and purging several times a day. She is having problems with occasional bleeding in the lining of her esophagus, her stomach is continually churning, and the enamel on her teeth is starting to erode. Because vomiting has become difficult for her at this point, she tries using laxatives instead, which worsen her digestive system even more. On some days she even gives up her beloved food entirely because of the abdominal pain she experiences whenever she eats. As a result, she has lost a fair bit of weight and people are starting to comment about it.

Do You Love an Addict?

If you're like most people who find themselves in relationships with addicts, you probably don't talk in depth with others about how you are feeling or what you are going through. You may be taking unnecessary responsibility for your loved one's behavior, feeling as if it is somehow your fault, and as a result you may be experiencing feelings of shame, guilt, and remorse. You convince yourself that the last thing you want is for anyone to know what is happening in your life, believing that no one would be able to understand. This can create a sense of isolation for you, because you may not realize there are other people in the same predicaments, experiencing exactly the same feelings you are.

Chances are you've tried many ways to change the situation, attempting to get some respite from the chaos in your life. The following are some of the most common tendencies of people who love an addict. Be aware of how many may apply to you.

* You are sick and tired of the pain and/or abuse in your relationships.

* You yell at the addicted person in your life, threatening to leave the relationship if the problem behavior doesn't stop.

* You complain to your friends and family members about this person even though you know that they don't know how to help you.

* You protect the addict by making excuses for the behavior.

* You make appointments with doctors and therapists for your addicted loved one, only to find that the person is unwilling to go.

* You try to convince yourself that the problem really isn't that bad.

* You feel sorry for yourself, baffled about why this is happening to you and what to do about it.

In addition, you may think the other person's behavior is your doing because you have not found a way to make the turmoil stop. Perhaps you feel like a bad parent or spouse because you think you should be able to do something to end this terrible situation. To make matters worse, your addicted loved one may actually be telling you that you are to blame for his or her addictive behavior!

"It's Not That Bad...Is It?"

If you have a practicing addict in your life, you may already be an expert in convincing yourself and others that the situation in which you find yourself isn't really that bad. You may have denial down to a fine art—in fact, this very denial may be the only way you can justify continuing to stay in the relationship.

You probably have your moments of despair, asking yourself why this is happening to you. Or you may have already become used to the pain and unpredictability, the feeling of waiting anxiously for your precarious house of cards to come tumbling down yet again. You likely live in a whirlwind of emotions ranging from fear, frustration, and hopelessness when things are at their worst, to relief, confidence, and a misguided optimism that all will be well when things are at their best.

It's even possible that you think it is normal to live this way—perhaps you believe this is how life is for everybody. You may already be so used to the lies, the deception, the manipulation, and the self-absorption of the practicing addict that living this way has become, in effect, your "comfort zone."

YES, IT REALLY *Is* THAT BAD!

But no one should have to live like that.

Although the details of your experience will undoubtedly differ from someone else's, the emotions you feel are often exactly the same emotions that other people feel when they are dealing with a loved one's addiction.

Some of the most common emotions include:

* guilt and shame

* anger and anxiety

* frustration and fear

* confusion and powerlessness

* hopelessness and depression

* desperation and despondency

If someone you love is abusing drugs or alcohol, or is engaging in other addictive behaviors such as disordered eating, problem gambling, smoking, Internet addiction, an abusive relationship, or compulsive over-spending, please remember that *there is hope for things to get better!* This book is going to show you how to do just that.

HELPING VERSUS ENABLING

Since it is likely that nobody has shown you how to improve your circumstances when dealing with a person with addictive behaviors, you probably don't really know what kind of action will truly help. If you are reading this book, it is probable that you have tried everything you could think of to be of assistance to your addicted loved one, likely to no avail. And, in fact, because you did not have any tried-and-true template to use, you may have been "enabling" the addiction to continue rather than helping it to stop.

When you enable other people, you unwittingly encourage them to continue their addictive behaviors. As an example, let's look at the case of a woman whose husband often drinks excessively at night, sometimes to the point where he is too hung over to go to work the next morning. If this is happening regularly, perhaps it has become her pattern to be the one to call her husband's boss and say that he is "feeling sick today" and unable to come to work. By participating in the relationship in this way and covering up for her husband, she is actually rescuing him and laying the groundwork for him not to have to take responsibility for himself. This constitutes enabling behavior on her part.

As she continues to shield her husband from the things he doesn't want to face about himself, she will likely find that she is developing some addictive behaviors of her own that may well be interfering with the potentially healthy functioning of her marriage.

For example, if she feels she needs to walk on eggshells around her husband for fear of setting off his anger, or if she believes that she is in any way responsible for her husband's drinking, she may not feel comfortable talking to him about the problems she is encountering in their relationship. Without this type of ongoing discussion between partners, issues that are already difficult to deal with will only become more problematic since neither person is taking any positive action to remedy them.

As we go through the top ten survival tips for loving someone with an addiction, you will learn how to offer healthier and more effective choices to your addicted loved one. When you are able to do this, you will feel a sense of realistic control in your life. This will also lead you to feel an increase in your self-respect, which is, without a doubt, the most important thing you can change about yourself.

FOCUSING ON YOURSELF

Your own recovery from participating in dysfunctional behaviors begins when you start to focus on *yourself*. In order to stay balanced and healthy while loving an addict, you must be willing to turn the focus of your attention and energy away from the addicted person and onto yourself.

As we go through the top ten survival tips together, you will be guided to look inside yourself to understand what you can indeed change about your life as well as what you truly cannot change. As a result, you will see some important shifts begin to occur in your significant relationships with others.

Perhaps the best news of all is that you will develop the increased self-respect necessary for you to feel happier and more confident in your most important relationship, the one you are in at all times: the relationship you have with yourself. As you gain control over your own life in healthy ways, you will ultimately become a role model for your addicted loved ones to gain control over theirs.

CHAPTER 2

Understanding Addiction in a New Way

There is nothing easy about loving someone who is actively engaging in any addictive behavior. In order to fully understand how to resolve the problems that arise from being in a relationship with an addict, it is necessary to first become aware of the nature of addiction. As you learn about what causes addictive behaviors and how they can manifest, you can then understand the best steps you can take to improve your situation.

Addiction in any form can make even the strongest relationships fail. People who are in the throes of active addiction are, essentially, completely self-absorbed. They are continuously looking for ways to get their next fix, whether it is the next opportunity to overeat, go shopping, gamble, smoke a cigarette, view porn on the Internet, or get high from a mind-altering substance. And, depending on the financial cost of their addiction, they may be always on the lookout for the monetary means, legal or not, to subsidize the behavior on a regular basis.

This leaves little time for addicts to focus on anything else, especially making an emotional commitment to the people in their lives. Relationships begin to unravel partly because the addict is not putting in the time and effort that are required to keep those relationships healthy and functioning well. When addicts are using mind-altering substances like alcohol or drugs, or engaging in mood-altering behaviors like compulsive shopping or disordered eating, they are so busy running away from their difficult emotional states that they are also not able to feel the joy and happiness that intimacy in relationships can bring. As well, closeness with others is shattered because of trust issues that develop when addicts lie, cheat, and steal from their loved ones. Addictions thrive in darkness: in order to keep his or her addictive behaviors alive, your addicted loved one will feel the need to remain secretive about them.

THE THREE FACES OF FEAR: WHY PEOPLE USE ADDICTIVE BEHAVIORS

All of us have certain behaviors we use when we are fearful of facing our emotional, spiritual, or physical pain, or when we feel as though we have no control over our lives. Of course, some addictions are not as overtly dangerous as others and, in fact, many are socially acceptable. But no matter how we attempt to hide from our reality, on some level we know that we're hiding. As a result of this inner awareness, our self-respect begins to suffer.

People who engage in addictive behaviors can be quite creative when it comes to their reasons for doing so. Most of the time, these so-called reasons are actually *excuses* for not wanting to feel the fear of facing what is really going on in their lives. Often, even when something relatively small goes wrong in the lives of practicing addicts, they prefer to escape from whatever it is rather than face it head on.

In order to do this, they find a behavior or a substance that will take them away from the difficult issue at hand. In the addictions field, this is known as a "broken shoelace" because something as trivial as that can be what leads an addict to engage in the chosen behavior. In this case, the addict's F-E-A-R really means **Forget Everything And Run.**

No matter what type of addiction people pursue, it will primarily be used *to change what they are feeling*. Most of the time, addicts use these behaviors to feel better about themselves and their lives. Instead of being willing to do whatever is necessary to attain a level of true happiness and serenity, they will opt for a quick solution to enable them to feel temporarily better.

On the other hand, there are also people who believe deep within themselves that they do not deserve to be happy; these are the ones who will sabotage themselves when good things happen to them. Those who have difficulty letting good things into their lives might decide to "celebrate" a happy event by going to the bar or to a casino or shopping mall. But ultimately they will likely end up feeling far worse because they allowed the addictive behavior to take over instead of being able to enjoy the happiness.

Then, based on faulty reasoning, they may then decide that life is unfair and nothing good ever happens to them. They might feel afraid even when they are experiencing good times, because they are convinced that something negative is waiting for them. People who respond to situations in this way are not looking at their lives realistically. When this happens, **F-E-A-R** can be defined as **False Evidence Appearing Real.**

When an addicted person decides to stop hiding from reality, however, anything is possible. Even a practicing addict who has been diagnosed with something as significant as a life-threatening illness could decide to use that situation as a springboard to stop engaging in the addiction and live with more integrity, in a more self-respecting way. If that person makes the decision to face reality head on, an addictive behavior will not be required. In this case, **F-E-A-R** can be translated into **Face Everything And Recover.**

WHAT IS ADDICTION, REALLY?

There are many schools of thought about what addiction actually is and what truly causes it. Most people who successfully participate in 12-Step programs such as Alcoholics Anonymous, Overeaters Anonymous, Gamblers Anonymous, or Al-Anon believe addiction has its roots in medical illness, considering it to be a disease. Believing that no real cure exists for the addiction but that recovery is possible one day at a time, they attend meetings and follow the prescribed 12 Steps of the program.

Other people wonder if perhaps there is a physical sensitivity to mind-altering substances that causes a person to feel "powerless" over the use of them. Because some people can experience toxic responses when certain types of drugs or alcohol are introduced into their bodies, they feel as though they are experiencing an allergic reaction to those substances, "losing control" when they ingest them.

As well, there has been much speculation (but no absolute scientific evidence at the time of this writing) about whether a genetic component factors into mind-altering addictions. If a genetic link to alcohol or drug abuse does exist, there would thus be a greater likelihood that addicts would turn to these substances if someone in their family of origin, or even in their extended family, has a history of substance misuse. However, this is not the case with all people who experience physical addiction to mind-altering substances. Although I became addicted to drugs and alcohol, for example, I do not have any history of that kind of addiction in my family of origin. Clearly, more research is needed before a definitive genetic link can be assumed.

Differences are noted with mood-altering addictive behaviors such as disordered eating, problem gambling, smoking, relationship and/or sexual addiction, and compulsive over-spending. When people indulge in these addictions, it is often because they have watched their role models, especially their parents, practice the same kinds of coping behaviors to feel better about what was going wrong in their lives. In this case, there would be no genetic component but rather a "do as I do" manner of avoidance. Arguments are ongoing as to whether these forms of addiction are a product of *nature* (biological, genetic) or *nurture* (environment, role model imitation).

Two essential hallmarks of addiction must be taken into account in order to have a full understanding of how addiction plays out: tolerance and withdrawal. *Tolerance* means that, over time, more and more of the chosen substance or behavior will be required to achieve and maintain the same effect. For someone using drugs or alcohol, it will not take long before the addict realizes that he needs an increase in the amount of the substance he is ingesting to reach the same "high." Likewise, for a shopping or gambling addict to continue to feel the desired effects of the behavior, additional trips to the mall or the casino will be necessary as time goes on. The same principle holds true for a bulimic person, who will binge and purge more frequently over time. However, an inverted tolerance exists for someone with anorexia, who will need to eat less and less in order to achieve the required result of marked weight loss.

Withdrawal refers to the discomfort addicts feel when they stop the addictive behavior. By definition, withdrawal involves a painful reaction that is always emotional and often physical, depending on the chosen addiction. The withdrawal of prolonged alcohol and drug use will often be physically severe in nature, while someone who has an Internet addiction or is codependent[1] in relationships will not generally feel the same kind of bodily discomfort. Whether the addiction is to a substance or a behavior, however, the withdrawal component will affect the addict emotionally, giving rise to such feelings as anger, fear, depression, and anxiety.

---

1   "Codependency" can be simply defined as putting other people's needs ahead of one's own, on a fairly consistent basis.

In truth, the addiction itself is actually a symptom of deeper emotional issues, precisely what the addict is trying to avoid dealing with and resolving. It is entirely understandable to want to feel good as much of the time as possible. However, when addictive behaviors are used to achieve those good feelings, there will be no healthy or lasting serenity. On the contrary, there can only be escalating problems. Learning to deal with the realities of life cannot happen when any type of "fantasy" is involved.

The only way to truly bring an addiction under control is to discover what caused it in the first place. It is never enough simply to treat the presenting addiction; in order to fully recover, it is necessary to develop the courage to go deeper. It is vital to discover past traumas and to heal any existing emotional scars that are still creating discomfort in the person's life.

The important work for you, however, as the loved one of an addict, is to develop your own self-respect. You need to learn how to stop enabling addicted people by becoming willing to allow them to find their own way and even hit bottom. This is what will lead them to choose recovery, and we will discuss this further in the chapters to come. It is not your job to help them discover their deeper issues; they may need the help of a trained professional to do that. If you find it difficult to detach with love, you may also want to reach out for professional assistance for yourself in order to get on with your own life.

TYPES OF ADDICTION: THE DIFFERENCE BETWEEN MIND-ALTERING AND MOOD-ALTERING

Although there are a number of similarities in the way addicts behave depending on their addiction of choice, unique patterns of behavior are associated with different forms of addiction.

One type of addictive behavior that people engage in is referred to as a *mind-altering addiction*. Chemical substances such as alcohol and drugs are used by people who wish to escape completely from their reality and feel what is commonly referred to as a "high."

When people engage in mind-altering substances, they generally are not able to maintain the efficient level of functioning that they can when they are not using them. People using even a small amount of heroin, cocaine, or methamphetamines, for example, would likely find it difficult to work while they are high, because these drugs would severely impair their logical and rational mental processes. They would be thrown into an altered mental state where reality and fantasy collide and, at times, they would be rendered unable to tell the difference between them.

Although people generally become cognitively impaired by using even a small amount of mind-altering drugs, ingesting alcohol may have a different effect depending on how much is consumed in a given period. For example, having one beer or a glass of wine with lunch during a business day might not have any strong or lasting impairment on one's functioning, nor will it blur the lines of reality and fantasy. However, if people consume several drinks at the same lunch, or if they are suffering from last night's hangover yet choose to consume even more alcohol, there will obviously be a more significant change in the level of functioning and perception.

The other type of addictive behavior people choose is known as a *mood-altering addiction*. This can include disordered eating, compulsive shopping and over-spending, problem gambling, smoking, sexual acting out, and ongoing codependency in relationships. Although these mood-altering behaviors do not create the same kind of physical or mental high as mind-altering substances do, they serve the same addictive purpose of providing relief from everyday reality.

As an example, let's delve a little further into the life of Janet, our compulsive shopper from Chapter 1.

> While beginning her routine of driving to the mall, Janet is focused on the thrill of her upcoming purchases. Upon entering her favorite store, as she has done so many times before, she is no longer thinking about the loneliness in her life. Janet enjoys chatting with familiar sales clerks as they give their opinions on what she is considering buying, feeling less lonely with each conversation. Her momentary joy feels so complete that she isn't even thinking about the vast amount of debt she has accumulated as a result of her ongoing shopping addiction. Her reality virtually eludes her as she enters into an altered state of momentary bliss, browsing through the merchandise, making her selections, taking out her credit card, and signing her name once again on the dotted line.

> Even as she carries her bags to her car and then into her house, Janet is still on her lovely vacation from her real life. She feels her customary emotional high from all the clothes and accessories she has purchased and, for just a little longer, all seems right with the world. It is only later, as she hangs her new items up in a closet already full of never-been-worn clothing items that still have price tags on them, that she begins to feel the familiar guilt and remorse she has felt so many times before. She then wonders why she bought even more things that she really does not need. She once again experiences a recognizable feeling of shame as she tells herself how foolish she was to have spent all that money yet again.

The major difference between mind-altering and mood-altering addiction has to do with whether the person's mental capacity is diminished. Either type of addiction will serve the same purpose of shielding addicts from their own difficult lives for a time. No matter which specific "behavior of choice" the addict in your life is pursuing, the emotional roller coaster and chaotic lifestyle will ultimately feel very similar for you if you love someone who chooses to remain in active addiction.

ADDICTION AS A CHOICE

Whether addiction is a disease, an allergy, the result of genetic programming, or a product of socialization, when a person engages in an addictive behavior, it ultimately stems from a personal choice to do so. Many people who are troubled by addiction admit that they make the choice to use the addictive behavior. Whether they settle on a mind-altering or mood-altering addiction, the bottom line is *they are making the decision to engage in a behavior that ends up causing them so much difficulty in their lives.* Although they make this decision initially to stop their pain, the ultimate irony is that, in every case, the pain only becomes worse as the addiction deepens.

This concept of choice may be more difficult to grasp when dealing with a mind-altering substance addiction. In 12-Step programs, Step 1 clearly states that addicts are powerless over their addiction, regardless of how that behavior manifests. If that is true, addicts may ask, how can using a mind-altering substance really be a matter of choice?

Here is the answer is to that question: Even if people do have an allergy or a genetic predisposition to a substance that makes them lose all common sense whenever they use it, they still have the choice about whether to use it in the first place. Millions of substance abusers consider themselves to have the "disease of addiction," yet they are able to recover when they *make the decision* to stop using.

Whether your loved ones have substance addictions, behavioral addictions, or both, and whether they are the result of a disease or a genetically inherited condition, addicts ultimately have a choice: they can either continue to engage in their addiction or they can stop. They may not be responsible for having become an addict, depending on a variety of circumstances, but *they are 100 percent responsible for their recovery from those addictive behaviors.*

The simple truth is that this is real for both addicts and the enablers of addicts. At the end of the day, all it takes is making the decision to stop.

Of course, this is almost always easier said than done. For most people, successful recovery from addictive behaviors takes some difficult inner work coupled with temporary feelings of discomfort. Some people are willing to do that work and feel that discomfort, while others are not. It's a choice.

People who are affected by a loved one's addiction also need to do their own inner work in order to learn how to stop enabling and start helping. If you love a person with an addiction, remember that you have your own comfort zone to find your way out of, your own addictive behaviors that you have probably been depending on for a long time. You will need to make the same decision as any other addict. If your choice is to become healthy and whole despite your loved one's troubles, then it's time to move on to the top ten survival tips for loving someone with an addiction.

CHAPTER 3

Survival Tip # 1:
Come Face-to-Face with Reality

"If nothing changes, nothing changes."

~ anonymous

We all know that, in life, some days can be harder than others. In fact, if you love an addict, your everyday life can be so difficult that the last thing you want to do is face the harsh realities of how bad things actually are. At times, all you may want to do is either scream and throw things, or cry your heart out in the corner of your closet.

Whatever form your loved one's addiction takes, caring about an addict can be a difficult and thankless job. You may be dealing with their unpredictability, never knowing when the next bout of outrageous and self-centered behavior is going to occur. Addicts are often in the habit of saying whatever is on their minds, without having the sensitivity to realize that what they say may be quite hurtful to those around them. That is why verbal abuse is so common in relationships with people with addictions.

The Jekyll-and-Hyde roller coaster of emotional instability can leave family and friends drained and exhausted. For example, you may not know when an alcoholic might be a "happy drunk" or a "raging drunk." Or you may not know when the next bout of sexual acting out will occur for a sex addict. This kind of unpredictability coupled with potential physical volatility in such relationships can result in anxiety, depression, and stress-related illnesses, as well as domestic violence and other forms of physical, emotional, or sexual abuse.

You may be spending a lot of your energy trying to run from the pain of your reality as it is, preferring to stay busy with other distractions that you feel you can deal with more easily. However, the problem is that these diversions, if left unacknowledged, can then wind up developing into addictive behaviors of your own. Although it is important to have activities you enjoy in your life so you are not always collapsed in the pain your loved one's addiction is causing, it is equally important to learn how to face your reality rather than run away from it.

Many adults who find themselves in relationships with addicts also had similar relationships as children. It is not unusual for a child of an alcoholic parent, for example, to grow up and marry someone with a mind-altering substance addiction. Perhaps you have never known anything other than dysfunction and addiction in your relationships; maybe you are doubtful that things could ever be different. It is important for you to understand that *you do not have to live this way.* There are alternatives to the pain you are experiencing right now.

SECRETS AND LIES

For most people who care about an addict, life is full of secrets. Not only is it difficult for you to accept the reality of your own situation, you also may not want anyone else to know about it for fear of judgment from them. And because most people do not talk openly about how hard it is to love someone who has an addiction, you probably have no idea of the huge number of people who are dealing with exactly the same issues you are confronting.

In your desperate attempts to hide from the truth of your reality and from the feelings of shame and guilt that truth may bring, you may not recognize that others in your life may actually be well aware of the problems you are dealing with, even if you have not told them. Also, because you imagine you have become so good at keeping secrets from others in your life, you may have become even better at keeping those secrets from yourself. You could wind up being the last to know of the severity of your loved one's addiction, or how transparent your suffering is to others.

Pretending that things aren't as bad as they are will not make them get better. Enabling people with addictive behaviors, as opposed to actually helping them overcome their addiction, makes the situation worse. Living in a fantasy space and hiding from the truth is not going to magically improve your circumstances. In reality, there is no such thing as magical improvement.

No matter which type of addiction a person chooses to engage in, loving a practicing addict guarantees that there will be dishonesty and manipulation in your relationship. Addicts need to set up their lives in such a way that ensures they have time to engage in their addiction of choice. Spending time with their loved ones is often not as high on their list of priorities, which can leave you feeling empty and unfulfilled.

As the lies are told and the promises are broken many times over, disappointments, betrayal of trust, and hurt feelings become the norm. In many cases, heated arguments will erupt in anger, even rage, as the addict tries to blame you for what he or she is actually responsible for doing. "If you didn't nag me all the time," the addict might say, "I wouldn't have to drink [use drugs, smoke, overeat, shop so much, spend all my time on the Internet, etc.] like I do." Of course, this is never true—it is just the addict's way of circumventing self-responsibility. But your fear of confronting the addict may be keeping you from speaking your truth. Unpredictable mood swings can make standard communication seem extremely complicated and problematic, and various types of abuse—physical, emotional, verbal, and even sexual—may arise, often developing into seemingly inextricable, negative patterns.

Everyone involved in these relationships suffers, as typical ways of relating are replaced with one unhealthy dynamic after another. Spouses, partners, parents, children, siblings, friends, and colleagues all experience varying amounts of stress when addictive behaviors of any sort are present. In short, life is hard.

Perhaps you have heard the saying, "Denial is more than a river in Egypt." If you are not facing your own reality, it is likely that you have developed another kind of addiction of your own: you could be "addicted" to denial or fantasy, pretending that things are other than how they really are. Or perhaps you have become addicted to the chaos and the drama so often present in these types of relationships. In either case, you may find yourself hesitant to shift out of the pretense so that you don't have to make any uncomfortable changes within yourself.

It is crucial to understand that when it comes to your own behaviors, your use of denial and fantasy can take on an even more menacing component. Making the choice to turn away from your reality will negatively affect your vitally important sense of self-respect. In the case of your addicted loved one, that decision can virtually spell the difference between life and death.

WAYS TO AVOID HARSH REALITIES

Addiction takes many forms, with a variety of consequences. Depending on which dysfunctional behavior your addicted loved one is engaged in, you may find yourself experiencing a constant, gnawing concern that you live with every day, wondering whether he or she is safe. Or you may find yourself being asked for money often and feeling guilty if you say no, worried that your loved one may resort to illegal means to find money as a result. Perhaps you feel you need to watch everything you say and do in order to "keep the peace" in your home, to prevent the addict in your life from becoming angry or violent. As well, you may be asked to do favors for the addict on a consistent basis, such as babysitting or running errands, and you may not know how to say no. If there are children involved, you may be justifiably worried on their account and want to intervene to assure their safety. The truth is that repeatedly saying *yes* to requests such as these does far more to enable addicts than to help them. But because you may be feeling utterly helpless, exhausted, or resigned, you may be choosing to simply give in to your loved one's demands, despite being aware of the consequences.

In order to avoid facing your difficult reality, you may have already discovered some of the following behaviors that *appear* to help you, as the loved one of an addict, get relief from your stress and make your life easier.

* **Denial** – the refusal to accept or acknowledge what is true. "Nothing is wrong, I'm fine with the way things are."

* **Rationalizing** – making up excuses for why your life is the way it is and why it will stay that way. In short, when you rationalize, you are in effect telling yourself *rational lies*. "He has such a difficult job and is under so much pressure that he needs to drink in order to relax" or "I can fix her if I just love her enough and do everything right."

* **Blaming** – diverting the focus of attention onto another person or situation so that you can avoid taking self-responsibility. "My partner doesn't appreciate how much I do for him/

her" or "If you would just get yourself together, I wouldn't have to nag you so much."

* **Self-blaming** – turning the feeling of blame inward and blaming yourself. This is often how codependent people and relationship addicts cope with their stress and sorrow. "I must be a terrible parent [partner, spouse, child, friend]. I must somehow deserve this kind of treatment."

* **Minimizing** – discounting the seriousness of your situation. "It's okay that he misses work sometimes because he is hung over—at least he still has a job" or "Even though she spends all her money at the mall, at least she isn't on the street doing drugs."

* **Anger and Hostility** – used to push people away when you don't want to deal with their questions or concerns. This technique is often used in tandem with other forms of denial. "What do you mean, I have to 'set boundaries'? Don't tell me how to live my life!" or "I'm doing the best I can, so leave me alone!"

* **Self-delusion** – convincing yourself that you don't really have a problem at all. "Why am I making such a big deal out of this? My life is fine the way it is" or "If I just love him enough, he will change."

Of course, it makes sense that you would want to avoid seeing the truth of the situation you find yourself in. Nobody in their right mind wants to feel pain, and this is the basic reason why people develop addictive behaviors in the first place. Ultimately, however, addiction in all its forms only causes even more pain.

Facing Reality

When you love a person who has an addictive behavior, it is easy to think you're already living in reality. Because life is already difficult and chaotic in that situation, you sense that if you don't keep your wits about you, things could easily get worse.

There is nothing pleasant about coming up against some of the issues that addiction brings. Why, then, would the number one survival tip be to come face to face with reality? Wouldn't it be better to simply find a way to pretend it's not really happening?

In fact, facing reality and coming out of the daydream that things will just somehow get better truly is the most important first step in surviving when you love an addict. It means accepting that parts of your life may be out of control as a result of loving someone who is engaging in addictive behaviors.

Many people with addicted loved ones feel as if they need to be the ones in control, particularly because addicts are notoriously out of control. If you are the spouse, partner, parent, child, or friend of an addict, it may be difficult for you to recognize that you are not in control of everything and everyone in your life. You may, however, actually find it easier to come to accept that truth than to continue living with the heartbreak that your fantasy of control has created. Making the decision within yourself to come out of that comfort zone can lead you to more peace and contentment than you thought was possible in your current situation.

The old saying, "If nothing changes, nothing changes," has stood the test of time for a reason. And right now, in this moment, the most important thing you can do is to recognize that you may be using a number of behaviors of your own to avoid dealing with your difficult situation—and to make a change by deciding to come face to face with your reality.

CHAPTER 4

Survival Tip # 2:
Discover How to Love an Addicted Person—and Stay Healthy

"People are like stained-glass windows. They sparkle and shine when the sun is out, but when the darkness sets in, their true beauty is revealed only if there is a light from within."

~ Elisabeth Kubler-Ross

Remaining healthy on any level—physically, emotionally, mentally, or spiritually—can be a challenge at the best of times. It is not always easy to find the balance we need to put that into daily practice. When we love someone with an addiction, however, this challenge becomes even more intense—and even more necessary.

Because addiction is tied into many dysfunctional and unhealthy ways of relating to other people and to the world at large, the concept of being healthy is often discarded, as you feel you are busy merely surviving your circumstances. But by no means does this have to be the case in your life!

Just as there are effective ways to deal with the addict in your life, there are also ways that are not only less effective but can actually be dangerous because they prolong the addiction. Learning to distinguish between them is necessary and will become vitally important to your self-care. Not only will you save a lot of time and energy when you relate to others in more self-respectful ways, but you will also witness much healthier results both for you and your addicted loved one.

One major skill you may need to learn or brush up on is setting and maintaining appropriate boundaries with the people in your life, addicted or otherwise. If you are having difficulty with that, it will be important for you to explore the reasons for your reluctance. As you understand yourself better on that level, you can then learn some assertiveness techniques to help you say *yes* when you mean *yes*, and *no* when you mean *no*.

JANNA'S DILEMMA

A bright and attractive twenty-eight-year-old woman with a good job, Janna had a number of close friends and an active life. Her partner of two years, Steve, liked going to the bar after work with his colleagues—often and regularly. Janna complained about this pattern many times, and she frequently asked Steve to come home after work instead so they could spend some quality time together. Rather than coming home, however, he began to ask her to come to bar with him. His rationale was that she would get to know his friends and colleagues and thus feel more a part of his social life.

In theory, this could be a healthy solution occasionally. But in this case, Steve was using manipulative behaviors with Janna because he actually had no intention of coming home most nights after work. Steve's plan was to continue going to the bar several evenings a week.

When Steve refused to take her complaints seriously, Janna decided to join him on a regular basis. In order to do that, she often found herself avoiding her own friends, whom she knew would disapprove of her decision. Gradually, she gave up the activities she had enjoyed in order to spend time with Steve in the bar. She also began drinking more than she previously had;

over time, she began to secretly wonder whether she might have an addiction to alcohol herself.

Janna knew she was not making healthy choices by accommodating Steve's wishes in this way, but she tried not to think about that. However, she was unable to stay in her denial for very long before her self-respect began to erode. She often felt hung over in the mornings, and the high quality of her work began to deteriorate. Janna didn't like how she was feeling physically or emotionally, but she feared she would lose her relationship with Steve if she caused any waves. As she became more frightened and clingy with Steve, he grew more distant and became increasingly critical of her. Janna found it increasingly difficult to rationalize and minimize the problems that her own dysfunctional behavior was causing.

To make matters worse, the emotional cruelty she was already receiving from Steve at home began to get worse: the more he drank over the course of the evenings they spent together in the bar, the more verbally abusive he became with Janna in front of his colleagues and friends. He would tell unflattering stories about her and began calling her nasty names like "idiot" and "slut."

Although Steve was actually embarrassing himself in front of his friends, Janna often found herself burning with shame. But because she was afraid of setting any boundaries with Steve, she tolerated his escalating behavior. In reality, she was quite intimidated by Steve's bad temper, but did not yet have any experience with speaking her own truth in such encounters. To try to make sense out of what was happening, Janna told herself that she somehow deserved such treatment; if she could just improve herself in some way, then Steve would stop behaving this way.

Janna had grown up with an emotionally and physically abusive alcoholic father who also made those kinds of comments about both Janna and her mother. Although she was not yet aware of it, this is what had created the foundation for her faulty belief that she must deserve this type of cruelty. She was so accustomed to being treated disrespectfully by her father, as well as by other men she had dated, that she did not even consider confronting Steve about his bullying behavior. Allowing others to abuse her in this way, and ultimately disrespecting herself in the process, had become part of Janna's comfort zone: although she did not enjoy being treated poorly, she was used to it and therefore "comfortable" with it. As a result, Steve was able to continue getting away with behaving badly without having to deal with any negative consequences.

Finally, Janna became so depressed and anxious that she found herself in jeopardy of losing her job. A negative review from her supervisor served as her wake-up call, and at that point she made the decision to face her reality. She reached out for help and, with the assistance of a skilled counselor, Janna was able to explore the reasons she was having such a difficult time setting boundaries with Steve. She also began to understand why she was allowing him to abuse her so often and so disrespectfully.

As her counseling continued, Janna's self-awareness developed and she began to learn more about herself. She could see how growing up with an abusive, alcoholic father and a passive, codependent mother had shaped her personality. She started to understand how this was influencing her life as an adult, appreciating the serious problems it had created for her. Although the dysfunctional dynamic had its roots in her family of origin, she came to accept that it was now her responsibility in present time to change her negative beliefs about herself.

Today, Janna no longer allows herself to be disrespected by anyone, not even Steve. Over time, their relationship has become much healthier: as Janna became stronger emotionally, Steve also decided to try therapy himself, realizing that he could indeed lose Janna if he did not change his ways. As a result, he no longer drinks every night, nor does he say abusive, demeaning things to her.

THE IMPORTANCE OF PERSONAL SELF-CARE

In addition to learning the importance of personal boundaries and how to set them, there are other necessary ways to keep yourself healthy while caring about an addicted person. *It is vital to look after your own life with holistic self-care* and to ensure a good balance with such things as supportive relationships, fitness, good nutrition, work or volunteering, and time for the fun activities that you enjoy. Even people with lives that are unaffected by addiction find it complicated at times to maintain that kind of balance. Although you may find it difficult to look after yourself in these ways while struggling with the problems an addicted loved one can create in your life, you will find, over time, that the rewards of doing so far outweigh the challenges.

When you are involved with a practicing addict, it can be all too easy to neglect your healthy self-care. You may find that you have become overly involved with your loved one's addiction. There are many ways to gauge this. For example, if you find yourself constantly obsessing about whether or how much your loved one is using or trying to come up with strategies that will make him or her stop the addiction, or if you are talking with people incessantly about the subject, you have likely crossed over the line into emotional dysfunction.

As well, you may be covering up for the addict, making excuses for the behavior with your friends and family, or lying to the boss about why he or she isn't at work today. In order to avoid conflict, some people even go so far as to enable addictive behaviors by giving substance abusers money to get the drugs or alcohol they crave, driving compulsive shoppers to the mall or gamblers to the casino, or bringing home certain types of foods that they know are potential triggers for their loved one's eating disorder.

A far healthier use of your time and your money would be to take the best possible care of *yourself* that you can. What the addict does or doesn't do is not in your control, but you can grab the reins of your own life by starting to take better care of yourself in a holistic way. However, if you are like many people who are in relationships with addicts, you may be so skilled in taking care of others that you have little or no idea how to even begin looking after yourself.

You can start by asking yourself a few important questions:

* Am I enjoying my life the way it is today?

* Do my relationships with others bring me fulfillment?

* Is the work I do satisfying and enriching?

* Do I have hobbies and activities that I enjoy doing on a regular basis?

* Do I take care of myself physically by sleeping well, eating well, and exercising my body?

* Am I looking after my emotional and spiritual needs?

If you have answered no to any of the above questions, it's time to step up your self-care. It is your responsibility to ensure you are living the life you want to lead. It has been said that *life is not a dress rehearsal.* This is your only opportunity to be who you are now, and it is your job to make your life as meaningful as possible for yourself.

JUMP-STARTING YOUR OWN SELF-CARE

Take some time to reflect on the questions above and answer them as honestly as you can. If your relationships are not fulfilling, perhaps you need to end some of them and reconnect with people you haven't seen for a while—or perhaps it would be good for you to meet new people. If you don't know how to begin doing that, try checking out courses offered by your local school board or community center and sign up for something that interests you.

You may not be happy with your job, feeling that it no longer fulfills you. If that is the case, you may want to explore some of your other interests to see if there could be potential work for you in those areas. If you don't feel as though you can leave your place of employment at this time, or if you aren't working right now, perhaps you could volunteer some time doing something you love, in order to nourish your soul and bring more happiness into your life. Making decisions to change or improve your circumstances will also contribute to increased self-esteem.

To feel as healthy and energized as possible as you begin to make some of these important life changes, be sure to take good care of your physical needs as well. Tell yourself the truth about the type and amount of food you've been eating and see if you want to make some healthier adjustments. If you have questions about that, a dietician or naturopath may be able to help you find answers. Perhaps you would benefit from an exercise program at a gym or fitness center; a qualified personal trainer could be a good way to start if you have been inactive for a while. Or you could begin to walk or cycle if you have been driving everywhere—getting out in the fresh air will help to reduce stress. Also be sure that you are getting restful, stress-free sleep. Let your physician know if you have been having problems sleeping, because there are often easy remedies for insomnia.

Last but definitely not least is the spiritual component of self-care. For some people, this might mean belonging to a specific church or spiritual community. For others, it might mean setting time aside to meditate, walk in nature, paint, or sing in a choir. This is a highly personal choice, and it means looking deep within yourself to discover what helps you feel joyful, nourished, and uplifted.

If you feel you need help putting any of these essential self-care pieces together, a skilled counselor or life coach will be able to assist you. Don't be afraid to reach out for help when you need it—this will actually be good role-modeling for your addicted loved one when he or she, too, becomes ready to make important life changes.

As you decide to practice healthier and more holistic ways of being in relationship with yourself, you will begin to see the ripple effects in all your relationships, including the one with the addict in your life. You will find that learning to develop your own sense of worth and value by treating yourself in ways that are more self-respectful will inevitably lead others to treat you with more respect as well.

Wouldn't that feel wonderful?

CHAPTER 5

Survival Tip # 3:
You Cannot Control or "Fix" Another Person, so Stop Trying!

"Never try to teach a pig to sing;
it wastes your time and it annoys the pig."

~ *Robert A. Heinlein*

Is it difficult for you to believe that you can't control another person—at least to some extent?

Like most people, you have probably tried repeatedly to change the behaviors of others in your life. Perhaps you have thought there must be a secret to this ability, and if you could only find it, then you could successfully make others behave the way you want them to.

YOUR GROWING-UP YEARS

Survival Tip # 3 tells you that you are not able to control another person. That is because it is absolutely impossible for you to control anyone other than yourself. Many of you will want to argue this point with me, but ultimately you will find that to be a waste of your time. No matter how hard you try to fight it, the truth still remains that you simply cannot control or change anyone else—it is only with the other person's agreement and permission that you will experience the semblance of control over anyone other than yourself.

The reason this may be difficult for you to accept is that, although they probably meant well, your parents, teachers, and mentors taught that you could, in fact, change or control another person. Actually, our whole society seems to have been built around that premise. As children, we were taught by our elders that we could control and change another person's feelings and, as we grew up, we became aware that by behaving in certain ways, our parents would either feel upset or happy with us. Our songs, television shows, and even the magazines we read continually informed us that we could indeed make a person love us if we would just look better, smell better, *be* better in some way.

You also may have learned at an early age how to best maneuver a situation so that you could get your own way, which could have led you to think you were changing or controlling someone. Perhaps your teary tantrums or angry outbursts scared other people and appeared to give you control over them.

For example, as a child trying to persuade Mom to let you stay up late when she wouldn't hear of it, you may have learned that if you cried or told her "I hate you!" she would give in and change her mind. Or if you wanted to borrow your best friend's favorite sweater even though she was resistant to that idea, you may have been able to persuade her by becoming insistent or by offering to lend her something of yours. Perhaps you became skilled at playing the guilt card on occasion, believing people would then do what you asked of them. Some of you may have even been able to convince a teacher to raise your B to an A by using some form of learned manipulative behavior.

Although these kinds of experiences may have helped you get what you wanted in childhood, they could have also caused some confusion for you as you grew older and found yourself in a world that does not actually exist. In the real world, you can't control anyone but yourself, and you especially cannot change an addicted person who chooses not to change.

To illustrate, what was the emotional effect on you the first time you discovered there was somebody whose behavior you couldn't seem to change? If you had an alcoholic father, for example, and you wanted Daddy to stop coming home drunk and belligerent yet he continued to do just that, how did it affect you to see that his choice to behave this way was something you could not control no matter how hard you tried? When you saw that you weren't able to change another person, after being erroneously taught you could, the confusion and despair you felt may have led you to believe that you just weren't doing things right or trying hard enough. Although nothing could have been further from the truth, the seeds of low self-esteem are planted in this way, as you begin to believe that you are somehow simply not good enough.

The fact is that we live on a planet of free will. We are all making choices every moment of our lives. Most people decide the course of their behavior on the basis of cause and effect, with the inherent understanding that whatever they choose will have positive or negative consequences. However, some people have no such acknowledgment of how free will really works, preferring instead to ignore potential results just so they can have what they want when they want it. People with addictions generally fall into that category.

Unlearning Old Behaviors

In order to benefit from Survival Tip #3, you will need to "unlearn" some dysfunctional behavior patterns and core beliefs you developed in childhood. It will be imperative for you to become willing to explore the possibility of having developed your own addictive behavior of trying to control others. In order to stop living in a fantasy and instead opt to be part of the world that actually exists, you will be required to control only yourself.

Let's look at your life today, as an adult. When you try to convince your partner, child, friend, boss, or anyone else do things your way, your success or failure depends entirely upon whether that person *decides* to do it your way. It is always the other person's choice. And the same is true of you—nobody can make you do something you don't want to do, because you will choose how you want to do things in your own life. In your adult life, even if someone is abusively attempting to coerce you to act in a certain way, you are still really choosing your own behavior. It all comes down to personal choice— yours as well as other people's.

This is how life is on a planet of free will: anything that has to do with anyone other than you is not in your realm of control. And although you may find it easier in the short run to choose not to believe this, that doesn't make it any less true, nor will that decision help your life in the long run.

The Serenity Prayer Can Help

If someone you care about is grappling with addiction, you may have been expending a lot of time and energy trying to change a person or situation that you simply cannot change. Once you can fully understand the difference between what you can and cannot change, life with your addicted loved one will become much easier.

The Serenity Prayer is a tool that may help you understand that there are things about your life you can control and change, as well as things you simply can't.

These days, many people have heard of the Serenity Prayer. Although no one seems to be sure who actually wrote this short but powerful piece, anyone who has attended a meeting of a 12-Step group such as Alcoholics Anonymous, Narcotics Anonymous, or Al-Anon for relief from addictive behaviors will recognize this prayer as the group recitation at the end of each meeting. The Serenity Prayer will provide you with an extremely helpful gauge to see whether you are trying to control people and situations that, in reality, you cannot control.

Let's take a look at the four lines of this prayer.

God, grant me the serenity
To accept the things I cannot change,
The courage to change the things I can,
And the wisdom to know the difference.

God, grant me the serenity…
Although the word "God" is used in the first line, alternatives such as Higher Power, Goddess, Creator, or Universal Force can also be used. Spiritual beliefs are very much a personal thing, and it is important to find your own way on that part of your journey. For example, rather than asking an all-powerful God to "grant" serenity, some people find it a better spiritual fit to say, "I want to have the serenity…" or "My intention is to develop the serenity…"

To have serenity means to have tranquility, calmness, or peace of mind. If you are not feeling a sense of serenity in your life, then your stress levels will be high. A lack of serenity will cause you to feel worried, anxious, and frustrated, and your physical and mental health will suffer.

…To accept the things I cannot change…
As we have discussed, although you may have believed that you can change another person if you just try hard enough, the truth is that we can't *make* anyone do something against his or her will. As human beings we ultimately have free will, and the only time people change anything is when *they make the decision to change.*

You always have choices as well, and one of your most important life decisions could be to accept the things—including the people in your life—you cannot change.

When you have chosen to see the reality of this concept, you will understand that you have no power over anyone who does not choose to give that power to you.

...The courage to change the things I can...
Now comes the hard part. You will need to come out of your own denial to fully acknowledge and accept that the only thing you can change is yourself—and then *make the courageous choice to do it.*

If you are in a relationship with an addict and have chosen to keep this person in your life, you may feel you are giving far too much of yourself emotionally and physically without getting much back in return. You might be angry with the addict for not giving you what you need, such as respectful behavior, and this could fill you with a variety of resentful thoughts. In simply trying to get some of your own needs met, you might even find yourself becoming emotionally manipulative with your addicted loved one.

Instead of attempting to "make" the addict change, a healthier choice would be to decide what you are and are not willing to put up with any longer and set clear boundaries. If those boundaries are crossed, or if you feel you are being treated disrespectfully on a consistent basis—which is likely when you are dealing with someone in active addiction—you then have the option to make more courageous choices for yourself, such as limiting or ceasing contact with the addict temporarily or permanently.

It will probably not be easy for you to take this kind of responsibility for yourself at first—and that is why this part of the Serenity Prayer calls for "courage." It doesn't take courage to do the easy things in life. It takes courage to be willing to change yourself if you are not happy with something in your life—a much more difficult goal.

It may indeed have been easier for you up until now to put all the blame squarely on your addicted loved one. But a different, more courageous choice would be to decide to look inside yourself to discover what your part might be, and to work on changing whatever dysfunctional behaviors you may be bringing to the relationship. It is only when we let go of our need to change other people and instead decide to change ourselves that we can truly begin to heal.

...And the wisdom to know the difference.
This last line is the most important part of the Serenity Prayer. When you have the wisdom to know the differences between what you can and cannot change, you will save yourself a lot of time and energy, because you will begin to concentrate on what is realistically possible rather than focusing on fantasies. You will stop trying to control what you absolutely cannot control.

In addition, when you start to set healthier boundaries with your addicted loved one, you will feel more respect for yourself. As you find yourself taking more personal responsibility for yourself and your own choices, you will also change the ways in which you allow other people to treat you.

Having the wisdom to know the difference between what you can and cannot change, and knowing how to change the things you can control, will create the serenity that you have been wanting to find in your life.

CHAPTER 6

Survival Tip # 4:
Stop Blaming Other People and Become Willing to Look at Yourself

"You must be the change you want to see in the world."

~ Mahatma Gandhi

It can be so tempting to blame someone else for our problems! Unfortunately, it is also a futile exercise because, when we blame another person, nothing really changes.

BLAMING IS A NO-WIN SITUATION

Blaming someone else for your lot in life essentially keeps you in the role of a "victim," believing you can be happy and at peace only when the other person changes his or her offending behavior. In truth, happiness is actually a choice we make in every moment. We can allow another's actions to detract from our serenity or we can decide to change what we can about the situation.

In addition, when other people feel they are being blamed, they often become defensive and less willing to make the very changes you want to see. As a result, situations continue as they have been, and negative feelings such as anger and resentment increase. When the temptation to blame another person arises, it may be time to ask yourself the popular question, "How has that been working for you?" More often than not, blaming somebody else is a lose-lose proposition.

It is true that other people's actions contribute to what is happening in our lives, as well as to our feelings about those circumstances. We are interdependent beings relying on one another every day for a great many things, seen and unseen; for example, in our society, most of us depend on others to make our clothes and grow our food crops. In our personal and work relationships, we are expected to treat others with care and respect, and we count on them to behave toward us in the same manner. Supporting one another in healthy ways is one of our best human qualities, and we all feel nourished and valued when we experience that kind of support from another person. It's a wonderful feeling.

Learn How to Support Yourself

If that supportive nurturing is not forthcoming, however, we can feel isolated and lonely. When we are not able to have our emotional needs regularly met from others in our lives, we tend to feel hurt and bitter. If this becomes the norm in your life and you are continually experiencing the pain of feeling unsupported, you can help yourself by taking a realistic look at how you might be contributing to that and what you can change so your needs can be met in healthy ways. Although this can be a challenge, as you learn how to look inward without feeling resistance, you will begin to see this as a wonderful opportunity for you to learn about yourself.

Doing this inner reflection will become even more important for you if the person you are depending upon for support is a practicing addict who, by definition, is self-absorbed. The addictive behavior becomes the significant relationship for that person and you, unfortunately, will most likely find yourself taking a backseat to it.

Understanding and accepting this reality is often difficult for anyone with an addicted loved one. It is especially hard when the addiction is a mind-altering behavior, because logic and reasoning simply don't work when people are drunk or high. Even when the addiction is mood-altering, such as an eating disorder, gambling, or compulsive spending, trying to challenge the addict about the problematic behaviors can feel like slogging through molasses.

Addicts have a tendency to blame others for their lot in life. They may blame their spouses, their bosses, their children, the weather, the proverbial "broken shoelace"—anything that will take self-responsibility off their own shoulders. Most people instinctively understand that pointing the finger at others keeps them from having to be accountable for their own behavior, and most addicts become quite skilled at playing the Blame Game.

Are You in an "Enmeshed" Relationship?

If you are a person who generally feels excessive guilt or who tends to take more than your fair share of responsibility, as many people who are in relationships with addicts do, then you and your addicted loved one will fit together quite nicely, though not in healthy ways. This is known as *enmeshment*, and you may find it quite difficult to extricate yourself from this sort of relationship.

As the loved one of an addict, you may unwittingly be contributing to the drama in the relationship. For example, you may be doing things such as regularly lending money to the addict in your life, yet feeling judgmental when that money is used to fuel the addiction. But if you don't approve of the way your money is being spent, perhaps you need to stop giving it to your loved one. In order to heal the painful dynamic of enmeshment, you will need to interrupt your old patterns of behavior and develop some new and healthier ways of relating to the addict in your life.

It is important to remember that denial is a strong component of addiction. When you attempt to deal with a challenging issue, the most natural response from the addict will be denial, defensiveness, and yes, blame. This will often leave you feeling unheard and alone in your misery, and you will undoubtedly be quite tempted to start projecting your hurt and fear onto your loved one. This is how blame manifests.

Coming from that very place of hurt and fear, it will be easy to tell yourself that if it weren't for the addict, your life would be great. If you could simply make that person stop using the addictive behavior, all would be well. But it is important to realize that, in some way, you have also been playing a part in this situation. In every relationship, it takes two to tangle and two to un-tangle. Although exploring your own dynamics can be a difficult road to choose, this very choice will ultimately lead you to the most satisfying result because, as you saw in Chapter 5, your own behaviors are the only ones you have any real power to change.

Another way you may be contributing to the dysfunctional dynamics in the relationship is with your willingness to always be a sounding board for the addict. You may be providing a soft shoulder where he or she can rant about the unfairness of life, even though you recognize that you never receive the same support in kind. The chances are that your addict will continue to vent to you for as long as you choose to be there to listen. If you are feeling somewhat like a doormat in your relationship, you need to look at what you are doing to allow that to happen. Continuing your negative patterns while blaming the addict will not bring about any healthy results. Instead, these types of situations will simply maintain the status quo and neither of you will have the opportunity to grow and change.

Hank and Laura Stop Blaming and Begin Healing

Hank and Laura were high school sweethearts who married at the age of twenty-three, a year after they both finished college. Ten years and two daughters later, they both worked hard to support their small family.

Everything seemed to be going well in their marriage until Laura discovered a chat room on one of her favorite websites. An avid reader from the time she was a child, Laura simply did not have the time to belong to a book club that met once or twice a month. When she discovered an online book club where she could, at her convenience, share ideas with others reading the same book at the same time, she was delighted.

At first, she would only go into the chat room once a week for a short time; however, as time passed, she gradually found herself becoming more engaged with the people she met there. As she grew to know some of them better, they began to talk more about themselves and their lives, in addition to discussing the book they were reading. She developed a friendship with a man named Rodney who lived in England and was also married. Because he was so far away from her home in Canada, Laura felt she could open up to him, sometimes sharing thoughts and feelings she had not shared with her husband. Although Laura did feel a little guilty about that, she rationalized it by telling herself that her friendship with Rodney was making her feel happier, which would only enhance her relationship with Hank.

But Laura's "rational lies" did not improve the relationship between them. Over time Hank felt her pulling away, spending more and more of her free hours on the Internet. He did not know about her friendship with Rodney at first, but knew something was amiss in their marriage. He tried to talk with her about his feelings, but to no avail: Laura would minimize his concerns so she could continue her secretive behavior with a man halfway around the world.

Hank repeatedly told Laura he wanted her to spend more time with him and with their children. Still baffled, he tried every-thing he could to make her see his point of view. One evening he accidentally discovered Rodney when he used Laura's com-puter while his own was being serviced. Pieces started falling into place and his wife's obsessive online behavior finally made sense to him. He made many attempts to reach out to her and make her stop what he believed to be an emotional affair. In his despair he pleaded and cajoled, then became sullen and angry. He inevitably confronted her with the ultimatum that he would leave her if she did not end her all-consuming online relationship with the man he now viewed as his rival. Hank was sure this would get Laura's attention and she would come to her senses.

However, Hank discovered instead that he was indeed power-less over his wife's choices. She ended up leaving Hank and her children, to the amazement of all who knew them. Laura rent-ed her own apartment and stayed there for several months. Eventually, Hank stopped trying to convince her to come home and instead began to focus on his own life with his children, who were suffering from the negative effects of their parents' enmeshed relationship.

Hank came to understand that whether Laura came home or not was ultimately her own decision. Although he was not happy about it, he knew that no one, including himself, could make that choice for her. One night, seemingly unexpectedly, Laura began to see the mess she had made of her life as well as the lives of her husband and daughters. She was aware that Hank was getting on with his life, and the thought of not being with him scared her. She decided to end her relationship with Rodney and focus her attention on the family she had been neglecting.

Hank and Laura both recognized that they had several pieces to put back together in their marriage, as there were now a number of major trust issues that needed to be addressed. With the assistance of a skilled couples counselor, they learned about their powerlessness over each other, and also began to see that this aberration in their marriage was not just Laura's responsibility. Each could admit there had been problems in their relationship they had not dealt with honestly, and this denial on both their parts had paved the way for the ultimate breach of trust that eventually occurred.

Today, Hank and Laura have a new respect for the fragility of a relationship. They understand that neither can control the other. Now they choose to allow time for individual decision-making as well as consistent checking in about the state of their marriage from each partner's personal perspective. They respect themselves and each other much more, with neither trying to control or change the other. And in a ripple effect, their children are learning to treat each other's decisions with respect as well.

HEALTHIER BOUNDARIES INCREASE YOUR SELF-RESPECT

The simple but difficult truth is this: if you are willing to put up with an addict's self-absorbed behavior without setting self-respectful boundaries, then you really have no one to blame but yourself.

In order for the relationship with your addicted loved one to transform into something more positive, you must first be willing to see how your own dysfunctional patterns may be contributing to the ve1y ᴏ.. lations you find untenable. You will begin to understand that *everything in your life begins with you* and ripples out from the relationship you have with yourself.

It is true that we teach people how to treat us: If you are not respecting yourself, other people will pick up on that and also treat you disrespectfully. It is your responsibility to start respecting yourself, to recognize the behaviors you are contributing to your dysfunctional relationship with the addict in your life, and to make the necessary adjustments. As you solidify your relationship with yourself, you may be surprised when other unhealthy and enmeshed relationships in your life also improve.

Maya Angelou offers this wonderfully sage guidance about self-responsibility:

> *If you don't like something in your life, change it.*
> *If the situation can't be changed, then change your attitude about it.*
> *Don't complain.*

The most courageous choice you can make is to stop blaming others and instead change what you can about yourself and your life. This is not always an easy task; please remember that it takes courage to do significant inner work. Many people feel they need some assistance at times from a skilled professional who can guide them on this all-important journey. If this is true for you, don't hesitate to find someone who will walk with you as you begin your path to self-respect and who will assist you in looking inward, making different choices, and transforming your enmeshed behaviors.

CHAPTER 7

Survival Tip # 5:
Learn the Difference between "Helping" and "Enabling"

*"We should not feel embarrassed by our difficulties,
only by our failure to grow anything beautiful from them."*

~ *Alain de Botton*

D o you feel compelled to help your addicted loved one? Are you afraid of what will happen if you don't?

Very little in life is more heartbreaking than watching people you love destroy themselves while in the grasp of addiction. It can seem so pointless for addicts to treat themselves this way, and as a loved one watching it happen, you will feel powerless—which, essentially, you are.

WHY YOU KEEP TRYING TO HELP

People who love addicts desperately want to help them overcome their destructive behaviors. They have experienced the devastation that addiction can cause and have witnessed their loved ones struggling and suffering as a result. Family and friends of addicts often feel anxious much of the time, and they are desperate to improve the situation they find themselves in: they want their addicted loved ones to recover physically, emotionally, and financially. If you are in this situation, you will likely be willing to do virtually anything to make things better. Unfortunately, even though you may mean well, you may not always give assistance in appropriate ways.

More than anything, as a loved one of an addict, you want the night-mare of addiction to stop. You may be tired of the anxiety you feel every day, worried about when the next argument will blow up or when you will be asked to do something you really don't want to do. You may sometimes fear for the addict's very life, and this trepida-tion may be with you on a daily basis, even in situations when the addict has not been in touch with you for a long period of time.

No matter what the details of the addiction are, you want the un-predictability of life as you know it to stop. Because you feel help-less, you often overcompensate for those powerless feelings by doing things you know you probably should not be doing for the addict. More than anything, you want that person to stop the addictive be-haviors and become "normal" again.

It is critical to understand the difference between *helping* and *en-abling* when you explore your options regarding how to assist an addict's recovery. As we saw in Chapter 1, your enabling behaviors, such as doing whatever is demanded of you whenever you are asked, will almost certainly lead an addict to continue engaging in the ad-diction. In contrast, a helping behavior, such as saying no when you mean no, will support the addict to develop the self-responsibility required to eventually stop the addiction.

CODEPENDENCY AND ENABLING

If your tendency is to enable, you probably find it easier in the short run to simply give in to other people's threats, manipulations, and mood swings. The idea of learning how to set and maintain healthy boundaries will feel scary for you, and you will worry that if you don't appease the addict, he or she may retaliate with even worse behaviors. In fact, many family and friends I've spoken with are ter-rified to set stronger boundaries, fearing that the addict in their lives will leave them or wind up on the streets. As a result, they choose to continually twist themselves into pretzels to make sure this doesn't happen.

Unfortunately, that is not an appropriate response to the situation; it ultimately does little if anything to help an addict stop pursuing destructive behaviors. For most addicts, the dynamic required for stopping an addiction is that they must reach some kind of "bottom." This means they need to see that they have something significant to lose if they continue to engage in the addiction. Some addicts need to lose a lot before they decide to abstain from their addictive behaviors. When they do not experience considerable consequences, many addicts simply continue on their path of self-destruction.

No discussion about the difference between helping and enabling would be complete without also addressing *codependency in relationships*. If you feel you are having difficulty overcoming your enabling behaviors, it will be important to understand how your own codependent tendencies may be getting in the way.

I like to use a simple definition: codependency is what occurs when we consistently put other people's needs ahead of our own. Another popular term for this behavior is *people-pleasing*, and many who are in close relationships with addicts fall into this category. In fact, the majority of people-pleasers are codependent in most of their relationships across the board, not only with the addicts in their lives. The following are some examples you can use to gauge your own codependency:

* You are tired of constantly giving to others in your life without getting much in return.

* You are concerned about the pain and/or abuse that you are experiencing in your relationships.

* You are extremely uncomfortable with confrontation; even when you feel disappointed, angry, or resentful, you do not admit this to others because they might become upset or angry with you.

* Rather than trying to change the dysfunctional dynamics in your relationships, you attempt to convince yourself that the problems you are experiencing are not really so bad.

* You feel sorry for yourself, baffled about why this is happening to you but not knowing what to do about it.

"BUT I'M SUCH A NICE PERSON!"

Because codependents consistently put others' needs ahead of their own, they often believe they are "nice" people.

"I'm doing what everybody wants me to do," you tell yourself, "so why do I feel disrespected by others so much of the time?" Indeed, this will be a real dilemma for you. As a people-pleaser, it will not make sense to you that you are being treated abusively by the very people you are trying so hard to accommodate.

Now, I'm not saying you're not a nice person. You probably do care about others and want the best for them. But the truth may be that you are not really as "nice" as you would like to believe, because, in fact, you're not saying *yes* to everyone else just to be kind to them. Nor do you do more than your fair share of tasks because you truly want to be of service repeatedly without any kind of reciprocal arrangement.

This may be closer to the truth for you: When you say *yes* (especially when you really want to say *no*), you are actually protecting yourself from having to face the potentially painful consequences that can result when someone is disappointed, angry, or frustrated with you for not agreeing to do what they want you to do.

As well, in order to feel safer, some codependents attempt to control certain situations that they find truly terrifying. For example, you may have found yourself actually assisting your addict to buy drugs, just to keep him or her out of dangerous circumstances.

MICHAEL AND JUDY: ENABLING VERSUS HELPING

Michael is a long-time heroin user. At the age of twenty-six, he has already been fired from a number of jobs and has lost the support of most of his family members due to his manipulative behaviors and unwillingness to receive treatment. He has been on the street for five years, sharing needles with other addicts and committing crimes such as theft and breaking into cars. He has often been arrested for these actions, yet is frequently let out of jail the very day he is taken into custody because of various flaws in the legal system.

The only remaining family member who will have anything to do with Michael at this point is his older sister, Judy. Michael sees Judy about twice a week when he contacts her to borrow money. When she connects with him, Judy consistently brings Michael food and lends him $20 or more. Although she is fully aware this money will be spent on drugs, she just can't bear it when Michael is upset with her. He has frequently accused her of not caring about him when she has tried to refuse his demands and, on occasion, has threatened to either leave town completely or kill himself when he doesn't get his way. Because she knows she is the last family member who will communicate with him, she is careful to give him what he wants.

Much to Judy's own dismay, there have been times when she has actually driven Michael to his drug dealer to pick up his heroin. She cringes inside when she thinks about this, and weeps whenever she admits it to anyone. More than anything, Judy wants Michael to stop using, but she tells herself the only way she can be sure he'll be safe, even alive, is if she "helps" him out.

This has been going on for several years. In his self-centeredness, Michael takes advantage of his sister's love for him as well as her fear of conflict. Because he is in active addiction, his life totally revolves around himself and his own needs. He does not see his sister's deep pain, and Judy does not divulge that to him. As a result, Michael has no need or opportunity to make a different decision. He does not see the need to stop his addiction or repair his relationship with Judy who, in her codependency, is now addicted to Michael's addiction as her life now revolves almost totally around him. In fact, because of the hopelessness, depression, and anxiety she feels on a constant basis, she is currently in jeopardy of losing her own job and her self-respect is at an all-time low.

The combination of Michael's ongoing heroin use and Judy's continued enabling behaviors have created a lose-lose situation not only for both of them, but also for their entire family.

WE TEACH OTHER PEOPLE HOW TO TREAT US

In order for codependency to be part of any relationship, two things have to happen: the people-pleaser has to say *yes* a lot more often than *no*, and the other person has to not only accept this but also begin to expect that to occur. Once this dynamic is in place, it can be difficult to break the cycle. Because codependents may actually be trying to protect themselves by side-stepping other people's anger and disappointment, which could be seen as a self-caring intention, it is unfortunately not a healthy form of self-care when it is done out of resistance to unpleasantness.

When you consistently say *yes* to another person, and when you accept any form of abuse as part of your relationships, you are essentially teaching those people it is all right for them to treat you that way. Although you might not be aware of it, you actually do have as much power and control as the other person does, because all of us can really only control ourselves.

When you *choose* to give your power and control to another person, you begin to feel the sting of codependency. The truth is that no one can disrespect you without your permission, and when you engage in people-pleasing behaviors, you are implicitly giving your permission to be taken advantage of and treated disrespectfully.

ARE YOU HELPING OR ENABLING?

When addicts are in the throes of their addiction, it generally takes a lot for them to be ready to stop. They have been using their chosen behaviors in order to escape from other issues in their lives such as unhealed traumas, difficult life tasks, or feelings that are uncomfortable to face. Their fear of not being able to engage in their familiar addictive diversions can be so overwhelming that they literally don't know who they are or how to relate to their lives without them.

But in order to become a healthy person physically, emotionally, and spiritually, we must learn to deal with discomfort and be willing to face our life tasks even when we find them to be unpleasant. When you allow the addict in your life to hide in addiction, you are not helping them. You are essentially "rescuing" them from taking full responsibility for themselves, which is not helpful to them at all. When enabled in this way, some addicts begin to believe they are not capable of taking care of themselves, which is simply not true. They have just not been called upon to do that, so they see themselves as incompetent. And the vicious cycle continues: the more they believe they cannot look after themselves, the more they will choose to use their addiction as a shield for the lack of self-respect they experience.

For a people-pleaser, the fear of confrontation can be overwhelming and will ultimately cause paralysis in your relationships. If this is a fear for you, then it is your responsibility to change that pattern. You may decide to receive some counseling to help identify what your fear is and where it originated. For many people, it stems from unhealed childhood trauma. Once you begin to understand yourself on a deeper level, it will become easier for you to set and maintain healthy, self-respectful boundaries in all of your relationships and, in so doing, you will be "helping" others by putting forth the expectation that they do their own inner recovery work. Can you see how it will actually be more loving in the long run to stop enabling your addicted loved one and start helping instead?

SHIFTING OUT OF CODEPENDENCY AND INTO HEALTHY ASSERTIVENESS

Now that we have established the difference between enabling and helping and you can see the need for a change in the dynamics of your relationships, you may be wondering how to start doing that.

Two things need to happen for you to be able to shift out of your codependency and into healthy assertiveness. As you saw, many people continue to enable in order to deflect other people's disappointment, frustration, and anger. Therefore, your first challenge will be to learn how to handle those feelings that others unload on you when you decide not to do whatever it takes to please them.

If you can deal with another's disappointment, frustration, or anger without being afraid of it, you can become emotionally free. If you can learn to stay true to yourself and make that your most important goal, you will no longer have to engage in people-pleasing behaviors because you will be able to assertively speak your truth. You will no longer have to live in fear.

When your addicted loved one demands something of you, it will become easier for you to tell him or her that what is being asked of you is not appropriate and you are choosing to not follow through with it. If the addict decides to rage or issue ultimatums, you will not have to give in to the manipulation. In short, you will stop enabling.

Your second challenge will be to increase your self-awareness. You need to be able to discern when something is a *yes* for you inside and when it is a *no*. If there are times when you are ambivalent or unsure about your inner feeling of *yes* or *no*, it is appropriate to tell other people you need to think about the issue at hand and will get back to them later with an answer.

This new behavior will require time and practice. When you begin, you may make a mistake and give in to an unwanted request, only later recognizing your error. But knowing you are working on developing this inner skill will help to prevent you from feeling so victimized when you find yourself still doing things you don't really want to do. You will know inside that you are in the process or making an important shift, and you will begin to feel some new self-respect—a concept that may have seemed foreign to you before.

Developing self-respect is an amazing journey. As you do your inner work and begin to make different choices, you will be amazed at the wonderful rewards that await you. The ripple effects are astounding. As you start to respect yourself, you will find you want to take the best possible care of yourself that you can. You will find yourself choosing healthier foods, wanting to exercise your body, and being more careful about the people you choose as friends. If you stay on this path, as a work-in-progress, you will find your entire life changes as your self-respect increases, choice by choice.

CHAPTER 8

Survival Tip # 6:
Don't Give in to Manipulation

"No price is too high to pay
for the privilege of owning yourself."

~ *Nietzsche*

It has been said that the least favorite word for an addict to hear is *no*.

When people with destructive addictive behaviors are not ready to make a major shift out of their addiction, they are virtually willing to do whatever it takes to be able to continue. To quote another slogan from 12-Step programs, practicing addicts "want what they want when they want it, and they want it right now."

Saying *No* to an Addict

When addicts who are determined to engage in their damaging behaviors are challenged by the people in their lives, they become master manipulators in order to keep the addiction going. Their fear of stopping is so great that they will do just about anything to avoid being honest with either themselves or with you. And when you find yourself on the receiving end of the drastic lengths addicts go to, you may not know how to handle it.

Some of the manipulative behaviors you may encounter when you say no to an addict will include lying, cheating, and raging, as well as blaming and guilt trips. Some addicts may also become depressed or develop other kinds of emotional and physical illnesses in an attempt to avoid dealing with life's responsibilities. All of these reactions can be difficult for you to deal with, especially if they occur regularly, so it may feel easier to simply concede to your loved one's demands. And that's exactly what the addict in your life is counting on, because that's the way the addiction can continue.

However, the problem is that the more you allow yourself to be manipulated by the addict, the more manipulative he or she is likely to become. People who want what they want when they want it generally do not give up easily, especially if they know from past experience that with just a little more coaxing, you'll cave in and give them what they want.

The following story shows how problematic life became when Andy's parents did not put a stop to his manipulations.

ANDY'S PARENTS FEEL POWERLESS

Bethany's adopted son, Andy, has a problem with alcohol. Now nineteen, he has been drinking almost daily since he was eleven years old. Andy had his first taste of beer when he was nine, and within two years his drinking escalated to bingeing on weekends with older teens.

Andy's birth mother was a heroin addict who lost her son to foster care when he was a toddler. When Bethany and her husband Paul adopted Andy at the age of five, they had no idea of the problems Andy had inherited due to Fetal Alcohol Syndrome.

During the past six years, Andy has had ongoing problems in school, including being suspended and expelled for fighting, stealing, and cheating on exams. He has stolen from his family as well in order to buy alcohol, and has lied to Bethany on many occasions about where he's been and what he has been doing. He has been in trouble with the law and has spent some time in a juvenile remand center. He adamantly refuses to participate in any counseling program at this time, and his parents feel powerless to force him to attend.

Andy decided to quit school without finishing eleventh grade. Now, two years later, he is depressed and having difficulty finding a job. He has no plans for his future. He lives at home, drinking and smoking pot in his room. Andy generally sleeps until mid-afternoon, and then stays up most of the night playing video games and continuing his substance addiction.

Paul does not condone this behavior and is at the end of his rope watching his son languish without direction. He has half-heartedly suggested they kick him out if he doesn't find a job "soon." His mother, however, wants Andy to continue living at home, no matter what. "At least I know where he is," she tells her husband. Although Andy is now collecting welfare each month, Bethany does not even think to ask him to contribute anything to the household financially because, when she has mentioned it before, he has become angry with her, and Bethany just can't bear that. As a result, there have been no consequences set for his lack of help around the house.

Andy rages and becomes unruly when he is challenged by either of his parents about the way he is living his life. Although Paul is able to deal with those reactions more easily than Bethany, he does not create any healthy boundaries for his son. For her part, Bethany has become so afraid of Andy's angry outbursts over the past few years that she just tries to keep things "pleasant."

Andy often spends his days at home, but at night he likes to go out partying with his friends. When he asks for money from his parents, Mom secretly gives it to him while Dad says no. This dynamic is played out frequently in their triad with most of Andy's demands. The result is that the parents are not united in their dealings with their son, which makes it easier for him to manipulate them.

It is not unusual for Andy to come home in the early morning hours, which contributes to many sleepless nights for his parents, who worry incessantly about him. When Andy does arrive home, he is often stoned, drunk, and loud. He has been known to cook himself a meal in the middle of the night, banging dishes, pots and pans, awakening Paul and Bethany, and endangering the household by cooking in that altered state of mind. He does not clean up after himself, and when they ask him to do that, Andy knows which buttons to push for the biggest emotional reaction. He swears at them, tells them what horrible parents they are, and storms off to his room, where he cranks up his music for all to hear.

Bethany and Paul love their son very much, even while they do not like many of his behaviors, and they do not know what to do to help him. One major problem is that they disagree about how to handle Andy. Because of the shame they feel about Andy's actions, Bethany coddles him while Paul scolds him on a regular basis. They have not spoken to a therapist about their situation nor have they attended any self-help groups. They are afraid to set any real boundaries with Andy, who now appears to have the most power in the household. Bethany and Paul both fear that if they provoke him too much, he might leave home and wind up on the streets—a thought that keeps them up at night with worry. They don't know what their options are and feel as if their hands are tied.

A Quick Review of Helping and Enabling

A quick review of the difference between helping and enabling is important here. When you allow addicts (or anyone else) to manipulate you, you are essentially enabling them to continue engaging in behaviors that keep them from developing both self-reliance and self-respect. This does not benefit anyone and is thus a lose-lose situation.

In order to respect ourselves, we need to have experiences that require us to handle life's complications. If you rescue others by enabling them, you rob them of the opportunity to learn how to deal with difficult situations. Because we develop our belief of ourselves as capable people by overcoming challenges, we need to encourage the ones we love to trust themselves and to learn how to handle the tough things in life.

Let's face it—life is hard for everyone at times. But in order for addicts to have the rewards of self-respect and self-trust, they have to learn how to do what life requires of them. And it is the same for you; if you let manipulation occur in your relationships, you are not requiring enough of yourself, and everyone will suffer as a result.

The truth is that none of us can be manipulated without our permission. Saying *no* is an important first step toward change—for you, as well as for your addicted loved one. Letting addicts know that you care enough to want a healthier relationship with them could be enough for them to understand that you're not trying to punish them by assertively maintaining your boundaries.

Once you have set the stage for manipulation in your relationships by implicitly agreeing to it, it may take a little while to change that dynamic. In the above example, Bethany might start by saying *no* to her son's demands for money, and perhaps pursue some counseling for herself to learn how to deal with Andy's anger as she makes this important shift out of her enabling behaviors. She might even decide to put the money Andy is asking for into a savings account that can be put toward his education or his first month's rent, when he is ready to become more responsible for his own life.

As you begin to set more appropriate boundaries and stick to them no matter how much others may try to dissuade you, the better chance you have of shifting out of a "victim" role in these relationships and into the self-respecting person you were meant to be.

CHAPTER 9

Survival Tip # 7: Ask Yourself the "Magic Question"

"Worrying is like a rocking chair: it gives you something to do but it doesn't get you anywhere."

~ *T. Harv Eker*

Sometimes we can become "addicted" to somebody else's addiction.

In the same way that addicts use drugs, alcohol, and other addictive behaviors to avoid dealing with their shame about feeling unworthy and unlovable, you may be concentrating too much on the addict's behavior to avoid having to focus on living your own life.

The Magic Question

Like many profound inspirations, the Magic Question is quite simple in nature but not always easy to answer: "How would my life be different if I didn't have this situation or problem?" If you didn't have the daily worries and anxieties of dealing with a loved one who is actively engaging in an addictive behavior, how would *your* life be different?

When I ask my clients this question, I sometimes receive a surprising answer, especially if they are able to go deeper than the obvious "My life would be great" type of reply. One man told me, "I wouldn't know what to do with myself," an honest response, and one that frequently traps people in their codependency. When our whole lives are centered on one particular problem or issue, the thought of no longer having to deal with it can seem frightening.

A woman answered, "I would feel useless," which showed that she was receiving her sense of worth or personal value primarily by being useful to other people. At that point in her life, she felt it necessary to *prove* she had value in the world, rather than simply knowing her own worth. As a result, everything she did for other people was in the guise of proving her usefulness. For example, she was starting to feel annoyed with her alcoholic husband but was still feeling a sense of her own value by playing out her roles of nursemaid and designated driver in their relationship.

When I asked another woman the Magic Question, she hesitated for a minute before answering. She then smiled sadly and explained that although she was growing tired of always having to plead with her Internet-addicted partner to spend more time with her and their children, she recognized that she was not yet ready to relinquish her full responsibility for the management of their home. The thought of not being able to use her partner's addiction as a method of maintaining total control in the family was, at first, terrifying for her.

When you are in a codependent relationship with an addict, you may be so used to putting his or her needs ahead of your own that you simply cannot imagine a different way of being. As you've seen in the last chapter about the difference between helping and enabling, this is not healthy for either you or your addicted loved one. It is a lose-lose situation that, in essence, helps no one.

Jack and Sally Clean House

Jack and Sally have been married for twelve years. Both in their mid-forties, it is the second marriage for each of them. Although they have no children, they have two dogs they both dote on and enjoy.

Sally has been a compulsive over-spender ever since she was a child. As a little girl, she would frequently accompany her mother, an over-spender herself, on exciting shopping excursions to malls and boutiques. Together they would decide on their purchases and proudly walk around with lots of shopping bags filled with goodies for themselves and everyone in the family.

Sally's most cherished memories of her mother revolve around those times together. During their precious shopping trips, Sally was able to forget about her mother's mental illness, much preferring the exhilarating ups of her bipolar condition than the agonizing downs when her mother rarely left her bedroom. Their special bonding occurred when her mother felt, as she described it, "on top of the world," but was blatantly absent when she was experiencing her "depths of despair."

As a teenager, Sally continued to love shopping. She often based her friendships with other girls on their willingness to frequently shop with her, as that was the best way she knew to emotionally bond with them. Early on, her bedroom felt like her safe haven filled with purchases that, although unnecessary, made her feel special and loved.

When Sally finished high school, she went on to study at a fashion college and became a buyer for a major retail store. In this way, she was able to fulfill her love of shopping by building her career around it. Not only did she begin to earn a large salary at a young age, she also received a substantial discount on what she bought in the store, allowing her to purchase even more items. Unfortunately, this only fueled her spending addiction.

Sally married her first husband Carl when she was twenty-two, and brought a great many boxes and bags of her own personal items into their new home together. It wasn't long before the clutter became more than Carl could deal with. When Sally refused to curtail her shopping, get rid of anything, or attend counseling, Carl left her and filed for divorce. Not even this turn of events was enough of a "bottom" for Sally; she simply buried her pain in more and more purchases.

Jack was totally smitten with Sally the first time he met her at a party several years after her divorce. She was pretty, well-dressed, and seemed like a confident woman. He didn't realize she had a problem with compulsive over-spending, and did not even wonder why she never invited him to her home. As a sales representative for a major computer firm, Jack was happy just to have Sally on his arm. Although he was successful in his career and earned a sizeable income, he had some self-esteem issues, often feeling as if he didn't deserve a beauty like Sally. Jack happily indulged her every whim, which suited them both well for a time. When they married a year later, Jack did not bat an eyelash at all the "stuff" Sally brought with her. In fact, he promptly bought her a bigger house in which to store it all and began to join her in the shopping addiction by making a number of expensive purchases of his own.

It wasn't long, however, before Jack grew tired of all his new toys. Their large home was fast becoming too small to house all of Sally's possessions. When Jack finally spoke up and questioned her about this, she became so angry and defensive that he dared not talk to her about it again. As a result, the combination of Jack's codependent enabling and Sally's unfettered addiction continued for many years.

Last year, Jack reached the point where he'd had enough of Sally's exorbitant spending addiction after discovering they were several thousand dollars in debt despite both of their ample incomes. Even worse for the extroverted Jack was that they had become virtual hermits in their home: nearly every inch of space was covered with clothes and other items Sally had purchased but never used, so friends were never invited to come over and socialize. Many of their friendships suffered as a result.

The ever-growing amount of clutter became so out of control that Jack no longer wanted to live with it. He began seeing a therapist who specialized in treating addictive behaviors. When she asked him the Magic Question, Jack was ready with an answer: "I would be able to enjoy my life and do the things I miss doing, like having friends over to watch the game on TV." After a brief pause he sheepishly added, "I might even be able to find my golf clubs."

As Jack continued with his counseling, he learned about Sally's addiction to compulsive over-spending. He also began to understand his own part in their unhealthy situation. Jack could see how he had been enabling Sally all this time by staying quiet, and how his fear of confrontation and abandonment had fueled his codependency.

Jack finally was ready for a different kind of life, one in which he could do some of the activities he enjoyed, such as hosting barbeques for his friends at his home or having extended family stay with him when they were in town. He no longer wanted to endure the stress of the financial debt they were

ing and, on the advice of his therapist, consulted a debt ounselor to begin developing a repayment plan. Lastly, but most importantly, Jack developed the courage to inform Sally that he needed her to get counseling for her addiction or else he would leave the marriage.

That was Sally's wake-up call. She loved Jack and did not want another divorce, which she could see was becoming a distinct possibility. She had reached the bottom with her addiction.

Sally and Jack have now been in individual and couple therapy for several months. They have agreed to hire a de-clutter specialist and are currently preparing to both sell and give many things away. As a result of their counseling, they have found other ways to bond aside from spending money, and Jack now speaks his mind with Sally. Today, their hard work has yielded them a strong marriage.

How the Magic Question Can Help You

If you recognize that you have been relating in codependent ways, you might benefit from an alternative wording of the Magic Question. Ask yourself instead, "How would my life be better if I wasn't consumed by behaviors that enable my loved one?" or "What would I have time to do *for myself* in my own life if I wasn't constantly focused on the addict?"

Once again, it is important to remember that you are powerless over anyone other than yourself. Try as you might to make others in your life behave differently, they will not make that choice until they recognize they have something of value to lose and become ready to make the necessary changes. And, of course, the same is true of you. As you begin to realize how fruitless it is for you to keep trying to change things that you do not have the ability to change, you'll gain the wisdom to know that what you can change is yourself and nothing else.

Altering your own problematic behaviors is as much of a choice for you as stopping full-blown addictive behavior is for an addict. It will probably not be easy for you to change your unhealthy patterns in the beginning, and will require both your courage and your determination. However, as you understand more about the numerous benefits of making the changes—especially the self-respect you will feel by making healthier choices—you will become more prepared to do the inner work it takes to begin to feel better about yourself and your life.

Asking yourself the Magic Question does not mean that you need to stop being concerned about your addicted loved one. Rather, it means developing a deeper understanding of the distinction between caring *for* others and caring *about* them. When people are not able to look after themselves—due to extreme illness, for example—then care-giving is indicated. But if you are looking after and trying to control people who actually can, and need to, look after themselves, you are care-taking or enabling them.

The one person you can and should be taking care of is yourself. Holistic self-care is a wonderful gift to give yourself and is the foundation of healthy relationships with others in your life.

Are you ready to make that shift into self-care?

CHAPTER 10

Survival Tip # 8: Know That "Self-Care" Does Not Equal "Selfish"

"What you want to be eventually, you must be every day.
With practice, the quality of your deeds
gets down to your soul."

~ Frank Crane

SELF-CARE—MY FAVORITE TOPIC

Practicing holistic self-care is the kindest and most loving thing we can do for ourselves.

Ironically, self-care is also an issue that meets with a great deal of resistance from many people. This is due to the common misconception that in order to care for and about ourselves, it is also necessary to selfishly put our own needs first at all costs.

For me, being self-caring and being selfish are two highly opposing ideas. To clarify, let's look at what happens when you travel in an airplane. As the plane is taking off, the flight attendant's voice comes over the loudspeaker. She makes her announcements about the safety procedures of the aircraft, advising that if you are traveling with children, infirmed, or elderly people, you should always put your own oxygen mask on first before trying to put anyone else's mask on them. On many flights, she will repeat her warning to never attempt to put someone else's mask on before putting on your own.

I see this as a perfect analogy of healthy self-care. It simply makes sense: if you cannot breathe yourself, how are you going to be able to help anyone else continue to breathe? In this case, it is not selfish to put yourself ahead of others. You must take care of your own needs first; only from there will you be capable of giving yourself to others who need your help.

The same principle holds true in your day-to-day self-care. The more you are looking after yourself and filling yourself up in healthy ways, the more energy and positivity you will have to give to others. You will find this to be true in all of your relationships; however, if you love a practicing addict, you can be sure that the majority of your healthy needs will not be met in that relationship.

Self-care is definitely an "inside job," which means that no one else can do it for you. Although it is true that other people may be kinder to you and treat you with more care and respect than you sometimes give yourself, it truly is *your* job to determine what your needs are. As well, you are ultimately the only one responsible for meeting those needs.

However, most of us do not learn this as children; self-care is often not something that was taught to us. We may have had parents, teachers, and other caregivers who knew how to take care of other people better than they knew how to treat themselves. As well, when we were growing up, our parents may have wanted to nip any childish selfishness in the bud, although they may have taken excessive measures in the way they tried to accomplish that. In many families, children learn that other people's needs and desires often come before their own. For example, "What will the neighbors think?" was a common refrain in my family of origin. In time, I came to believe that my needs did not matter as much as my neighbor's needs, and I carried that faulty core belief well into my adulthood with staggering physical, emotional, and spiritual costs to myself.

Today I understand that I am the center of my own universe, as indeed we all are—and that is the way it is *supposed* to be. This does not mean I have license to hurt others just to please myself. What it does mean is that it is my responsibility to know what my healthy needs are and to make sure they are met, just as it is your responsibility to do the same for yourself.

THE PEOPLE-PLEASER'S CREED

For those of us who grew up to be people-pleasers as a result of our family's belief systems, shifting out of that identity can be a struggle. It is, however, a challenge that will bring tremendous rewards into your life on many levels. If you would like to make that shift for yourself, it will be helpful to first understand the dynamics at play.

As you learned in Chapter 7, people-pleasers rationalize their codependent behaviors by telling themselves what "nice" people they are. They do their best never to hurt anyone else's feelings in an attempt to get everyone to like them. However, they do this not because they are nice, but because they want to avoid conflict and other types of unpleasantness at all costs.

Codependency thrives in an atmosphere of apprehension. In order to shield themselves from the dreaded negative emotions of those around them, people-pleasers do whatever they can to make other people feel comfortable. In essence, they twist themselves into pretzels in their quest to have everyone like them. The people-pleaser's creed is *"I must never hurt another person's feelings."* Therefore, if anyone has to feel hurt in a given situation, people-pleasers choose to bring that upon themselves rather than risk someone else's anger, judgment, or disappointment.

Remember that codependent people consistently put others' needs ahead of their own. Even as they rationalize their unending pleasantness, they rarely acknowledge that this kind of inauthentic behavior leaves them feeling victimized by others much of the time. They fail to recognize that *we teach other people how to treat us*: by behaving like victims with no self-caring boundaries, codependents are setting themselves up to be treated like doormats by the very people they wish would care about them. This dynamic becomes confusing for people-pleasers, who often have great trouble understanding why others are abusive with them when they are so nice!

If you have people-pleasing tendencies, chances are you are uncomfortable in any situation you consider to be emotionally disagreeable. A major part of your personal self-care will need to include learning how to deal with the very unpleasantness you fear so much. As you discover methods that work for you, your fear will gradually diminish and you will become free to be your authentic self in any situation—and this is the most wonderful, self-respecting gift you can give yourself.

The Self-Care Creed

As you might expect, the Self-Care Creed is quite different from the People-Pleaser's Creed. To be truly self-caring, you must be willing to put your own needs first when that is appropriate. Instead of always worrying about what others are thinking of you, your first concern will be about how you are feeling about *yourself*, using your healthy sense of self-respect as your gauge.

My father was fond of saying "You wouldn't worry about what others think of you, if you knew how infrequently they do." It was somewhat crazy-making for me to receive this message at the same time I was being told I should be concerned about what the neighbors thought, so as a child, I could not make much sense of my father's proclamation. Today, however, I understand that other people are busy living their own lives as the center of their own universes. My

job is to live in a self-respecting way, to the be
day at a time. My job is to be proud of myself a
way I am living my life.

The Self-Care Creed is

*"Although I care about other people's feelings,
the way I feel about myself is most important to me."*

When you are following the Self-Care Creed, you are setting beneficial boundaries with others in your life, including your loved ones. Even when this feels difficult, you assess the need for healthy limits by asking yourself the following question: "What do I need to do in this situation, or what do I need to *not* do, in order to feel good about myself?"

Shifting from the People-Pleaser's Creed to the Self-Care Creed involves three specific actions. First, you need to give yourself permission to be uncomfortable for a while as you're changing your responses toward yourself and others. Second, you will be required to be more gentle and patient with yourself—please remind yourself that becoming skilled at something new takes not only time but also courage. Third, you will need to practice your new behaviors repeatedly to begin to feel more confident and self-respecting. In doing this, you will begin to experience the amazing ripple effects of healthy self-care.

The Difference between Self-Care and Selfishness

Many people get these two ideas confused. You may be thinking that if you adopt a practice of healthy self-care, putting yourself first, you are being selfish. Although it is possible that others could perceive you that way and accuse you of selfishness, if your self-care is holistic and self-respectful, that will not be true at all.

ishness basically means that you want what you want when you want it, and you are willing to step on whomever you have to in order to get it. That actually sounds more like the behavior of the self-absorbed addict. If you are in a relationship with a practicing addict, it is more probable that you have been trying to take care of that person's needs ahead of your own. As you have continued to do this on a daily basis, you have no doubt begun to feel depleted, exhausted, and resentful.

It is important to understand that the addict in your life has an investment in your continued codependency. Remember that people use addictive behaviors in order to get away from having to take responsibility for themselves—they want you to take care of them so they don't have to. As soon as you begin to change your problematic patterns and start taking better care of yourself, your addicted loved one may begin to use even more manipulative behaviors to stop you from growing and changing. Accusing you of being selfish may well be part of the plan to keep you in line. If you know this ahead of time and are prepared for it, your shift into self-care will be much easier.

To be *self-caring* means that you respect yourself enough to take good care of yourself in all areas of your life, to the best of your ability. In a sense, when you are practicing healthy self-care, you are being *selfish* because you are giving to yourself, but it is not with the same kind of self-absorption that constitutes the negative form of selfishness.

As you start taking care of yourself and feeling the self-respect that goes along with that, you will find your energy returning. From a more grounded and centered place, you can then decide whether the people in your life actually need your help or whether it might be better for everyone if you pull back and allow them to find their own way. Not only will you be able to assist others without enabling them, but you will also become a positive role model for practicing healthy, holistic self-care.

The Four Areas of Holistic Self-Care

As we saw in Chapter 4, stepping up your self-care will bring more ease and serenity into your life. In order to become as self-caring as possible, it is essential to look at all four elements of holistic self-care: physical, emotional, mental, and spiritual. To neglect any one of these areas will cause an imbalance in your overall health. Some of these components may overlap, while others will be separate and distinct. Let's take a look at each of the four aspects with an eye on what you might choose to improve in your own life.

Physical Self-Care
This aspect of self-care will include anything that has to do with our physical bodies, addressing healthy eating, exercising regularly, sleeping well, and maintaining our overall physical health and well-being.

You have probably heard the saying "You are what you eat." People who follow healthy eating patterns generally make similar food choices, such as a variety of fruits and vegetables, whole grains, proteins such as lean meats, legumes, fish, and soy, and a decrease in dairy products. For snacks, they will often select items that are low in sugar and empty calories, such as nuts and nut butters, granola bars, and baked potato chips or vegetable chips. Many health-conscious people will choose organic foods when they can afford them.

However, most people with even the healthiest diets allow themselves to have occasional treats like desserts, chocolate, and salty snacks. The trick is to do this in moderation in order to keep food sensitivities under control. If you try to completely deprive yourself of the foods you love the most, you could find yourself engaging in addictive patterns like secretly bingeing and purging in order to satisfy your taste buds or to change your feelings of resentment about not being able to eat your preferred goodies. It is usually not necessary to rob yourself of your favorite foods unless your self-control becomes an issue or your food allergies make this problematic. That being said, if you feel like you are an emotional overeater, or if you're not eating enough, your self-care may also involve working with a skilled counselor who can help you understand what is causing you to go to one extreme or the other with food.

Another part of physical self-care is, of course, exercise. I know some of you may be cringing as you read this, but exercise can mean anything from going to the gym three or more times a week, to walking ten to thirty minutes a day.

It is important to *meet yourself where you are* in terms of what your body will be able to handle. If you have been active all your life, then running, cycling, or working out several times a week may not be a problem for you. If, however, you have been sedentary for a long while, or if you have struggled with illness that has hindered your physical activity, you may want to start with simple stretching each day, then walking for just a few minutes as soon as you feel up to it. Perhaps you enjoyed swimming or dancing in the past and would like to try that again now. No matter what form of physical activity you choose, your body will thank you for the least little bit of movement, and your self-respect will increase because you will know you are taking care of yourself in a significant way.

Another important part of physical self-care is making sure you are getting a good night's sleep regularly. Although mild insomnia is common occasionally for most people, if you are experiencing any ongoing sleep issues it would be wise to consult your family physician, as many symptoms can easily be remedied. Sleep deprivation can result in a number of negative consequences, such as lack of concentration, irritability, loss of appetite, and emotional unrest, so it will be beneficial for you to get this condition checked out.

As you increase your physical self-care and begin to feel healthier, you may find yourself looking at some of the other addictive behaviors you have been indulging in, to see how ready you are to let go of any of them. For example, are you drinking more than you'd like to be? Are you smoking cigarettes?

When I started taking better care of myself physically, I began to find it difficult to continue my fifteen-year, one-pack-a-day smoking addiction. I had tried to quit several times over the years and was unsuccessful. But as I began to practice healthier self-care, I became more aware of the poisons I was voluntarily putting into my body, and I was no longer able to feel good about myself when I lit up a cigarette. My fledgling self-respect was finally starting to feel more important than continuing a destructive, expensive addictive behavior. Although it was difficult for me to stop smoking after all those years, I felt so grateful to at last be ready, and at that point, it was actually much easier to quit than I thought it would be.

No discussion about physical self-care would be complete without also talking about the more enjoyable aspects. Perhaps you are fond of looking for bargains in vintage clothing stores or going for leisurely weekend walks with your beloved dog. When was the last time you treated yourself to a facial, or gave yourself a manicure or pedicure? Perhaps your hair would look good with a new style or some highlights. Have you been experiencing a healthy sexual relationship with someone you care about? It's important to have fun with your self-care and not just focus on what you "should" be doing. Enjoy yourself!

Emotional Self-Care

Practicing emotional self-care means that you are looking after yourself in ways that help you feel grounded and balanced. No one feels wonderful all the time, and it is not unusual to have difficulties in life. However, we need to ensure that we don't allow ourselves to get stuck in negative emotional patterns that have become comfort zones for us. In order to counteract this, we must take care of our emotional health.

When you are feeling emotionally healthy you will find yourself feeling calm, centered, easy-going, and friendly, with the ability to feel grateful for what you have in your life even if things are not perfect. On a sunny day, you may notice how beautiful the blue sky is and on a gray day the sound of the rain on your window may enthrall you.

Emotional self-care is a wonderful gift to offer yourself. It is a win-win situation because not only are the results rewarding, but the process can also be a lot of fun.

Think about it: when was the last time you enjoyed an afternoon with a nurturing and supportive friend? How long has it been since you set some time aside to read that book you've had on your nightstand forever? When did you last do some journaling about yourself and your life? Have you perhaps found a counselor or mentor who can help you understand your life when things feel a little crazy for you? Are you making time to enjoy a good meal or to play a swift game of tennis? Or perhaps what you need more than anything else is some time alone, to explore your inner feelings and do whatever activities feel right to you at the time.

Some people are more easily able to understand the potential pitfalls of not practicing healthy physical self-care than they are attuned to the possible risks of faulty emotional self-care. This is because the physical body often begins to show signs of neglect sooner than the manifestations of poor emotional well-being become evident. But if you are not taking care of yourself on an emotional level, many problems can also arise.

Symptoms of emotional distress begin for most people as a sense of generalized irritability. You may not know exactly what is going on for you internally, but you feel somehow "off"—just not like yourself. When this goes on for any length of time and is not addressed, increased nervousness and anxiety usually follow. Feelings

of depression, helplessness, guilt, shame, and emotional a,
other possible results of not following a plan of emotionally
self-care.

Behavioral manifestations of this kind of emotional burnout will
also begin to show up in your life. These may include being late more
often than you used to be, experiencing increased absenteeism or
poor performance at work or school, becoming more judgmental of
others, gossiping about people, and chronic complaining. You could
find yourself becoming more defensive or pessimistic, with an overall intolerance of other people beginning to show. As this occurs, you
may prefer to engage in solitary activities such as excessive reading,
watching too much television, or spending inordinate amounts of
time on the Internet. It is also possible that instead of facing the fact
that something is amiss in your life, you could choose to stay very
busy and socially active, preferring to lead a life of constant activity
and even chaos to avoid having to deal with the mounting emotional
stress you're experiencing.

For each person, emotional self-care may look a little different, but
the key element in being able to look after yourself in this way is
self-awareness. In 12-Step programs, a helpful acronym you can use
when you are not feeling quite right emotionally is **H-A-L-T**, which
stands for **hungry, angry, lonely, tired.** You may not always know
what is contributing to your emotional confusion, but this gauge can
assist you in determining the kind of self-care you need at any given
time.

As soon as you become aware of feeling uncentered emotionally, try
asking yourself what you need at that moment. The following questions can help:

* Am I *hungry*? Is my blood sugar low, do I need to eat something?

* Am I *angry*? Is there an emotionally frustrating or difficult situation in my life that I need to address and resolve?

* Am I *lonely*? Do I need to reach out for some connection with people who care about me? Do I need to schedule a get-together with a friend or have a date-night with my partner?

* Am I *tired*? Do I need a nap right now? Am I getting enough sleep? Am I handling my everyday stresses in healthy ways?

* Is there anything else I may be overlooking right now in terms of taking better care of myself?

Using **H-A-L-T** as a yardstick for your emotional self-care can help you pinpoint what you need in the moment, allowing you to feel better more quickly. You'll know you are experiencing emotional health when you can handle life's many ups and downs, even when you feel challenged and perhaps overwhelmed by them. As you begin taking responsibility for this aspect of your self-care, emotional health will follow as another wonderful ripple effect.

Mental Self-Care

It is also our responsibility to keep our minds sharp. As we age, and as we experience difficulties in our lives, our minds will begin to show signs of decline. An example of this could be having more bouts of the "What did I come into this room for?" syndrome than you used to. To continue to have healthy and active mental abilities, we need to engage in activities that support our mental and intellectual well-being.

From their research over the years, many neuroscientists are now telling us that our brains are like a muscle—use it or lose it. More and more, brain researchers are promoting the development of a mental self-care plan. The following are four components for more robust mental health:

* Keep your activities *interesting*.

* Make sure that some of your mental activities are *communal*.

* Take advantage of *new technology*.

* Stimulate your mind with *brain-teasers*.

Some of the *interesting* activities you pursue can include reading (both fiction and non-fiction), writing a daily blog, or doing cross-word puzzles. If you are mathematically inclined, you may enjoy Sudoku, bridge, or backgammon. Chess and scrabble are also engaging games that will keep your mental juices flowing. Learning about a foreign country's culture and language will help to keep you mentally sharp. And studies have shown that learning to play a musical instrument has a similar effect of stimulating your brain.

Your mental health will also benefit from *communal* activities with other people such as attending classes or a lecture series, playing cards or board games, and engaging in stimulating conversation. These social pursuits do not have to be limited to your peer group; you can also learn and have fun with your children and grandchildren, or you can volunteer at a food bank or local hospital.

To take advantage of *new technology*, just look at some of the latest extraordinary gadgets on the market. For example, many of the newer cell phones will do a vast variety of tasks, such as allowing you to surf the Internet, answer e-mail, or even download a full book to read page by page while you're in line at the market, in the doctor's waiting room, or stuck at the airport. Most people already have access to a computer. If you feel you're not computer-savvy and would like to learn more, you might enjoy taking a class at your local library to learn how to use basic computer technology such as Internet and e-mail—a whole new world awaits!

Brain-teasers are puzzles and riddles that tickle your brain and help you to think outside the box. There are many different types of brain-teasers, such as visual illusions, memory games, and logic problems to decipher. Some are interactive and can be done on the computer, while others may be fun to do alone or to share with other people. You can find some examples of brain-teasers at http://www.sharpbrains.com/teasers. Enjoy!

Just as physical exercise will help keep your body toned and supple, challenging yourself mentally on a regular basis will keep your mind in good shape, potentially protecting you from such conditions as Alzheimer's Disease as well as simple long-term and short-term memory loss. As you can see, staying mentally fit is indeed an essential part of any well-rounded self-care plan—and it can be fun to implement.

Spiritual Self-Care

This fourth aspect of holistic self-care will help you identify your heartfelt values and beliefs as well as understand more profoundly how you perceive your purpose in life. Spiritual self-care guides you in discovering the deeper essence of yourself as a human being, assisting you in taking the best possible care of yourself on all levels.

When we can see life as a spiritual journey, our difficulties often become easier. For some people, the term *spiritual* might have religious significance, while for others it may have more of a mystical connotation. Simply put, a "belief" is something that makes sense for you; therefore, whatever meaning you ascribe to a spiritual path will be right for you.

Perhaps your family of origin brought you up in a particular religion. If your choice has been to continue practicing in that faith, you may find your spiritual meaning in a church, temple, mosque, or other religious center, participating in daily or weekly services and classes. On the other hand, some people whose family practiced a certain religion make the choice not to continue in that same belief system. If that is the case for you, perhaps you have already found something that has more meaning for you in your life today.

For instance, you may feel your spirit come alive by studying about the Law of Attraction or some other alternative to organized religion. Maybe yoga gives you the relaxation and peace of mind you are seeking. Perhaps you would enjoy going to meditation classes with other like-minded people, or it could be that meditating at home is more of a fit for you.

Many people also find their spirituality in nature. Perhaps going for long, peaceful walks or sitting by the water listening to the crashing waves or a gurgling stream can fill you with a deep sense of awe and respect for the mysterious beauty of the world. Whatever it is that makes you come alive on a spiritual level is what you must pursue, for that is what will keep you excited and on track. Without it, life simply does not feel the same.

A final note about spiritual self-care: To be truly spiritually healthy, we must be able to embrace our inevitable uncertainty as part of our understanding of ourselves. As human beings, there are a great many things we can never know for sure, with questions of a spiritual nature being high on that list. Many people try to find certainty instead because they believe they will feel somehow safer if they can explain the unexplainable. I prefer to honor my doubts when they come up, knowing that feeling doubtful is part of the human condition for all of us.

Rather than trying to comprehend the incomprehensible, we need to understand instead our own individual belief system, remembering that a belief is simply what makes sense to each of us. Despite our doubts, we can strive to live with the faith that we are already "safe" spiritually, no matter what happens. It has been said that fear and faith cannot co-exist. I believe that; it makes sense to me. Therefore, if indeed they cannot co-exist, then I must choose between them. Although I feel fearful and anxious occasionally, just like every other human, my choice is to live primarily in faith, trusting the beliefs that enrich my life and nourish my spirit. I invite you to seek and discover what makes you joyful and juicy spiritually, and to live your life according to those beliefs.

PAMELA TEACHES JASON HOW TO TREAT HER

Pamela is a fifty-nine-year-old woman who now feels as though she is in the prime of her life.

This wasn't always the case. Pamela's son Jason has been addicted to crack cocaine for the past seven years. Before he discovered crack, Jason had abused marijuana and alcohol regularly. He was also addicted to watching porn and playing video games on the Internet. Jason neither worked nor attended school, preferring to spend his days pursuing his addictive behaviors. Well into his mid-thirties he still lived with his mother, paying no rent and contributing virtually nothing to the upkeep of their shared home.

No matter how Pamela begged, pleaded, and cajoled, Jason adamantly refused to give up his addictions and would not see a counselor for help. This pattern went on for many years with Pamela, a single mother, finally crumbling under the weight of all the stress involved in loving an addict who was choosing to remain unhealthy.

In desperation Pamela finally went to see a therapist herself, ostensibly to find out how she could help Jason. Fortunately, the therapist she chose had a background in addictions counseling, working with loved ones of addicts as well as the addicts themselves. With her guidance, Pamela began to see that the methods she was using with Jason had actually been enabling him to continue his many dysfunctional behaviors. She concluded that she would need to make some major shifts in the ways she was dealing with having an addicted son. The most important change she made was to begin a holistic self-care program. Regardless of what Jason chose for his own life, Pamela started to deeply understand that she had a right to a happy and fulfilling life, and after years of struggling and suffering, she found she enjoyed the process of putting those pieces into place.

Perhaps for the first time in her life, Pamela developed a caring relationship with herself. She began eating food that was more nutritious and exercising her aging, overweight body. As difficult emotions came up in the course of her own therapy, she learned how to honor them without blaming or shaming herself. As time went on, she joined a meditation class and began attending yoga several times a week, meeting like-minded people and forming new friendships.

Within a year of starting her own therapy, Pamela's weight decreased and her body had changed so much that she needed to purchase a new wardrobe, much to her delight. Her social life was thriving, and she met a man with whom she began a romantic relationship. This was all very new for her, having devoted so many years to looking after Jason's every need.

What Pamela did not expect, however, was the immediate and volatile reaction she received from Jason when she took control of her own life. Almost overnight, as it seemed to Jason,

Pamela began to leave her son to live his life as he chose, and she stopped nagging or pleading with him to change his ways. She left the house every day to pursue her own interests, no longer shopping or cooking for him, no longer cleaning up after him. Jason resented this turn of events and became furious when he realized that something quite significant had changed in their relationship. His behavior toward his mother became at first subtly more abusive, with nasty, derisive comments said under his breath about her different friends and activities. But before long he was yelling at her and calling her names, creating a lot of unpleasantness in the home they shared together.

As a result of her therapy sessions and the support groups she was attending, Pamela began to understand that beneath Jason's anger was a hurt and scared little boy. He was worried that his mommy would no longer provide for him and he would have to actually grow up and take responsibility for himself. With her therapist, Pamela explored her own past choices of allowing her son's addictions to dominate their home life, as well as her options regarding what she could do if she wanted to change that now. Gradually, Pamela realized that allowing Jason to get away with treating her disrespectfully was not helping anyone: that choice was both enabling her son and leaving her feeling badly about herself.

Pamela understood that if she did not set appropriate boundaries with Jason, she was essentially teaching him that it was all right for him to treat her badly. "If you choose to continue that kind of relationship with him," her therapist asked, "what incentive does he have to stop his abusive behavior toward you?"

Pamela had to agree that this was a good point. She decided to learn how to set assertive, healthy boundaries with her beloved yet troubled son. His resistance and continued abuse soon brought her to her "bottom" with her own codependency, and she told Jason that he would have to leave her home and find somewhere else to live. Although Jason was astonished and tried to test his mother's boundary several times, it did not take him long to leave, especially after Pamela threatened to call the police if he did not go.

Pamela and Jason subsequently struggled through some difficult times together. However, Pamela chose to continue her journey of recovery; she knew she needed to stop her own codependent reactions to Jason's addictive behaviors. As Jason watched his mother become holistically healthier, her strength served as a model of what he also could achieve. After many years of living as an addict, Jason eventually decided to seek therapy himself. He successfully completed a three-month residential treatment program and has been clean and sober for two years as of this writing. He continues to deal with his addiction to the Internet, but he is able to hold a job and is planning to return to school to become an electrician.

The relationship between mother and son is now much more appropriate and healthy. They see each other often, but they also now have their own lives with their own separate friends and activities. Pamela will no longer tolerate any kind of abusive behavior from Jason and, as a result, he has become less angry and antagonistic with other people as well.

Although Jason and Pamela's story has a happy ending, it is vital to understand that even when we change our lives for the better, there is no guarantee that our addicted loved ones will also choose to follow a healthier lifestyle. We must make these changes primarily for ourselves, not for anyone else. If we adjust our behavior only to motivate other people to alter theirs, we are once again trying to control other people, which, as we've seen, does not work.

Because Pamela decided to reach out for help for herself and learn how to practice consistent, holistic self-care, she not only changed her own life but also paved the way for her son to make that choice as well. Even while loving her addicted son, she was finally able to see that her own sanity was at stake because of the many years she had spent trying to change someone other than herself. When she realized she was, in fact, addicted to the chaos that Jason's addiction caused in their lives, she chose to begin living her own life in a much more self-caring and self-respecting manner. The icing on the cake, for Pamela, was that her son ultimately chose to do the same for himself.

CHAPTER 11

Survival Tip # 9: Rebuild Your Life

"That which we persist in doing becomes easier—not that the nature of the task has changed, but our ability has increased."

~ Ralph Waldo Emerson

ACCEPTANCE AND SERENITY COME FIRST

As someone who loves an addict, you know the devastating toll addiction can take on families and other significant relationships. You understand, first hand, the frustration, anger, fear, and confusion that accompany your deep and sincere concern for your addicted loved one. You also inevitably live with shame and guilt as you wonder what you might have done wrong to make this circumstance occur in the first place.

Hopefully, as you've been reading the preceding chapters, you've begun to see that all these feelings are normal in this situation—everyone who goes through this feels the same way to some extent. Even more importantly, my hope is that you realize there was nothing you did to create someone else's addiction. Engaging in addictive behaviors is, without exception, the choice of the person who is behaving in that particular way. Even if your actions have not been altogether healthy in the past, that will not be enough to *make* another person become addicted to dysfunctional lifestyle choices. There are, of course, other ways to deal with problems that occur in life and within any given relationship without resorting to dangerous and destructive activities.

As well, by reading this book, you have no doubt begun to understand that you are completely powerless to change your addicted loved one. Until people *want* to transform their lives, change does not happen no matter how hard you might try to make those shifts come about. That particular sense of powerlessness is possibly the most difficult aspect of all for the loved ones of addicts to come to terms with. However, once you can truly accept that, ultimately, you can do nothing to make your addicted friend or family member hear the voice of reason until they are ready to do so, you are ready to achieve a sense of serenity.

More often than not, both this acceptance and serenity precede the possibility of rebuilding lives that have been shattered by the throes of devastating addictive behavior, both mind-altering and mood-altering. Once the feelings of acceptance and serenity are experienced, you can begin to establish a healthier life for yourself. This will not mean that you no longer care about your addicted loved one. Rather, it means that instead of depleting huge reserves of energy trying to control another person, you can now use that same energy in more positive ways to take back control of your own life.

THE NEED TO REBUILD AND THE COURAGE TO CHANGE

Once again I am reminded of one of my favorite sayings: *If nothing changes, nothing changes.*

This simple statement explains a profound truth: Until we change something, our lives basically remain the same. All of us know that changing anything can be difficult. This is especially true of transforming something about ourselves. If we look again at the Serenity Prayer, we are reminded that the third line says, "The courage to change the things we can"—and we have now established that the only thing we can truly change is ourselves. All of us are courageous when we choose to change what is not working in our lives.

I like to use the analogy of a baby who is just learning to walk. From where he is sitting on the floor, he pulls himself up with his chubby, underdeveloped little arms to a standing position. As he looks around from this perspective, he decides all is well and embarks on his first step. That goes well, so he decides he will take his hands off the coffee table he has been using as support.

Oops! In a split-second, he finds himself on the floor once again—and now he has a decision to make. Will he sit there and cry, refusing to ever get up again? Will he scream in frustration because things didn't quite work out the way he wanted on his first try? Or will he look around, perhaps even laugh at himself as he becomes acclimatized to what has just happened, then lift himself up and try again?

This baby's choices are akin to the decisions you will have to make, time and again, as you develop your own courage to change. When you can look at your life honestly, you will come to understand that if you have been in a significant relationship with a practicing addict, your coping strategies have probably not given you the desired result of changing that person.

If you are ready to live a new kind of life, you will need to make some potentially difficult choices. But remember that in order to alter any type of dysfunctional behavior, *you must first be willing to sit in your own discomfort* without trying to medicate yourself in any other ways. Once you have made the decision to try and try again, like a little child learning new skills, you will feel uncomfortable for a time. However, the good news is that making these healthier choices will send your self-respect skyrocketing, and you will be able to pat yourself on the back for the courage you are displaying.

Won't that feel better than continuing to live as you've been living?

How To Begin? Try Some Baby Steps

I can hear some of you questioning, "Yes, but how do I begin to rebuild my life?" If you're even asking that question, you are well on the road because you have accepted the importance of doing it!

The best way to come out of your own entrenched addictive behaviors, such as enabling and people-pleasing, is to focus on your own self-care, *one baby step at a time.* Rebuilding your life will bring you a greater sense of happiness and fulfillment, and it is your most important overall responsibility. The time to start the transformation is in this present moment. As the saying goes, "If not now, when?"

The marvelous thing about baby steps is that they do not remain first attempts for very long. In fact, by starting slowly, your small efforts actually open the floodgates for so much more to come into your life. But instead of becoming overwhelmed with all of that too quickly, baby steps allow you to become accustomed to your achievements more gradually and help you to develop your new sense of yourself over time.

To begin the process of rebuilding, let's look again at the concept of holistic self-care, which we discussed at length in Chapter 10. If you feel unfulfilled in any of the four aspects we examined—physical, emotional, mental, and spiritual—you can begin to transform your life with baby steps by exploring the kinds of things that might fulfill you.

Physical Baby Steps

What would it feel like for you to be more at ease in your physical body? If you have been low on energy lately, what could you do to pep yourself up? Perhaps a first step would be a ten-minute walk in the fresh air once or twice a week. If you enjoy music, try taking your iPod or mp3 player with you so you can listen to your favorite tunes at whatever volume you like. If you love being in nature, you can focus instead on the trees, birds, and flowers around you. For those who have exercised before on a regular basis but have let it slide, a small step might be to go back to the gym or out for a run a few times a week.

The idea with using baby steps is to first assess where you are with your current self-care and then raise your personal bar just a bit. Expect a little more from yourself, but not more than you can handle. Be realistic about your self-expectations or you could set yourself up to fail, and there's no reason to do that. Just meet yourself where you are and start from there.

For example, perhaps your weight has become an issue and you would like to do something about that. Think about what a first step could be for you. Are you ready for a weight-loss program such as Weight Watchers or Jenny Craig? Or would it be better for you at this time to start by drinking more water and less soda each day? If you use your intuition and listen to your inner voice, you will more than likely know what you need to do to begin your physical self-care.

It will be wise to contact your doctor if you have been having trouble sleeping or if you are experiencing any difficult physical symptoms. Although for some people the thought of having a full medical checkup can be somewhat daunting, doing just that could either put your mind at ease or show you what you need to know to become healthier. Maybe you have let your important dental health slide. If so, a first step may be to call your dentist and schedule an assessment of what is needed.

If you feel close to being ready to stop smoking, or if you feel you may have been drinking too much lately, a positive initial step could be to use the Internet to look for groups with meetings that could assist you with cutting back or quitting completely. Once you have that information, see if you can raise your personal bar a little higher by actually attending a meeting or two, either in person or online.

It is generally accepted wisdom that ignoring a problem does not make it go away. And remember—if not now, when?

Emotional Baby Steps
Emotional self-care is about examining your feelings and learning how to express them in more appropriate ways. Taking care of yourself emotionally means looking within so you can better understand the choices you've been making, as well as the reactions you've had to situations you've found yourself in. Once you have a better grasp on that, you can learn how to transform the negative energy of emotions that have kept you stuck in your old dysfunctional ways into more positive energy that will help you to achieve your goals.

For many people, taking care of their emotional self-care may seem like a daunting task. To keep yourself from feeling overwhelmed, you will again need to identify some baby steps to start with. One gentle, effective way to begin taking stock of your emotional life is to write a gratitude list each night before you go to sleep. The beauty of doing this is that if you know you'll need to come up with five to ten things you're grateful for every evening, you will actually begin to look for those things as you go about your day. Doing this will create a different, more positive energy for you, as you focus less on what isn't working in your life and more on what is going well. Although the items on your gratitude lists will at times overlap, it's a good idea to try to vary them while looking for new things to feel grateful about. Give it a try for a week and see if it works for you—it may become a habit you'll want to continue.

Another tool I enjoy using to maintain and increase my own self-awareness is journaling. Writing about my thoughts and feelings helps me feel more "present" with myself. It's as though I'm opening my head and letting my ideas, emotions, theories, and opinions fall onto the paper where I can actually see and make some sense of them. I often suggest that my clients keep a journal of what happens for them during our sessions, because it provides a useful tool for them to be able to look back at their own growth during our time together. If you choose to journal as well, you can either use your computer or write in a book of your choice. (Many bookstores carry a large selection of lovely journals to choose from.) Either way, you may find that journaling helps you increase your emotional self-awareness as an adjunct to the thinking or talking you're already doing.

As your emotional self-awareness develops, you will find yourself feeling more energized, more alive, and less numbed-out. As we've already discussed in Chapter 10, it is also vital to include some fun activities in your emotional self-care, and your new-found vigor will empower you to enjoy them even more. Another first step in this area could be to make a list of some things you like to do, creating a balance of both social interests and more solitary pursuits. Such a balance is important because there will be times when your friends or partner will be available and other times when you'll feel like being alone. For example, you may enjoy seeing movies in a theater, and it would probably be more fun to share that activity with a friend or loved one. If you like to sing, you might enjoy being part of a choir; in that case, you could find out what kinds of choirs are in your area. At other times reading, playing the piano, or cooking a gourmet meal may appeal to you, all of which would be more solitary endeavors. Having that combination of activities to do on your own and with other people will contribute to a healthy, well-balanced life.

When beginning to rebuild your emotional self-care, you may want to consider finding either a counselor or a life coach to assist you. A counselor/therapist will help you make sense of the feelings you are experiencing as you move from your "old" life into your new one. He or she can suggest additional ways of dealing with difficult or painful emotions that could be keeping you stuck in your dysfunctional behaviors. A life coach will provide you with fresh approaches to the more practical aspects of rebuilding your life. The difference between these two roles is that a counselor or therapist can at times also act as a life coach, guiding you with contemporary and innovative suggestions, while a life coach often may not be qualified to assist you with the deeper emotional issues you may be experiencing at this point.

Mental Baby Steps
Your mental baby steps will relate to maintaining your brain's strength and resilience. In Chapter 10, we discussed a variety of methods to do this, and to ensure that your mental activities are interesting, communal, fun to do, and up to date with the latest technology. Going back to your list of favorite things to do, which among them might be most stimulating for your brain? Sometimes it is good to "stretch" yourself mentally and do things that require a challenge. For example, if you enjoy movies, you could rent a foreign film that requires you to read subtitles while also watching the story unfold onscreen. Reading mysteries or watching them on television may also be mentally stimulating, especially if you have a tendency to try to solve the puzzle before the end of the story.

If you enjoy playing cards or board games with others, you may want to check with your local community center to see what they offer in terms of bridge classes or ongoing scrabble games. Perhaps you've been longing to learn a new language as an adjunct to planning a well-deserved trip abroad. If you feel you need a smaller step before actually attending a class, you could go to your public library or bookstore and pick up a how-to book for that particular language. Once you decide you really do want to continue learning, you can then sign up for the class.

Learning about new technology is another way to exercise your brain muscles. If you're already familiar with basic computer functions such as e-mail or surfing the Internet, maybe you could learn how to take photos with a cell phone and then upload them to your computer. You will then be able to e-mail them to family and friends who do not live nearby, creating a fun way to stay in touch. You might even discover that you enjoy photography and decide to pursue that interest. Like several other first steps, this one could lead to classes in which you would meet like-minded people you might enjoy getting to know. All of these activities will serve as building blocks for reshaping your life.

Spiritual Baby Steps
Spiritual baby steps will help you bring your deeply held beliefs into alignment with the life you're living. They will also assist you to begin to discover what those beliefs and values are, if you have questions or doubts about them.

As you saw in Chapter 10, *spiritual* can mean different things to different people. This term may have religious meaning for you, or it may relate to such activities as meditation, yoga, or spending time in nature. How you see yourself spiritually will determine your first steps as you rebuild that part of your life.

If a more formal, organized religion is something you'd like to have in your life but have been neglecting for a while, reconnecting with the denomination of your choice will be important. An initial step could be to contact a friend you've known from the same church or temple and become reacquainted, or you may simply want to attend a service with people you already know there. If you're not sure which church or temple would suit you, perhaps you could call a few and ask some questions to assess which might be a good fit.

These days, you have many more alternative spiritual choices. You can choose from churches such as Unity and Celebration of Life, which offer services and classes that discuss ideas like the Power of

Now and the Law of Attraction. If you feel more alignment with those spiritual concepts and would like to be part of a community, you could go online and see if anything similar is available where you live. Some websites also provide online chat rooms and sharing sessions. Why not see what you can find?

Being part of a spiritual community is not important to everyone. Perhaps nature is something you derive great pleasure from; in that case, going for long walks in the woods or near the water could be just what you need to be able to clear your mind and find some answers to your life's most challenging questions. When rebuilding your spiritual life, it is important to learn how to nourish your soul and give yourself what you need on that level.

BELLE'S BABY STEPS

Belle and Liza are sisters. Only two years apart, they were close as children, especially because their single mother often left them alone together while she was working. In recent years, however, they have had problems in their relationship resulting from Liza's gambling addiction.

Liza began playing bingo when she was a teenager, accompanying their mother weekly to the bingo hall. While there, she would watch as her mother's moods shifted depending on whether she won any money. If Mom won that night, things were wonderful: she would be kind and accommodating, buying gifts for Liza and her sister. But if Mom lost, things became scary for Liza as her mother would rage and become verbally abusive toward her. Although she disliked these behaviors in her mother, she found herself putting up with them because the "highs" were worth it.

Over the years, Liza continued her gambling, moving from bingo to slots to horseracing and finally graduating to blackjack, both online and at various casinos in her city. When she married and had her own children, she found herself taking her shifting moods out on her family, just as her mother had done with her. Liza did not like the fact that she was repeating her mother's dysfunctional behaviors, but she felt powerless to stop. Both her gambling and her resulting reactions seemed to be out of her control.

In personality and temperament, Belle was different from her older sister. While Liza squandered her time and money gambling, Belle pursued her education, finally graduating as a social worker with a specialty in child protection. In her professional life, she was required to set many firm boundaries and make a lot of difficult decisions regarding child apprehensions from parents who were abusive or negligent, and she had little trouble doing that. In her personal life, however, things were quite different.

As a registered social worker with a knowledge of addictive behaviors, Belle tried for many years to make her mother and her beloved older sister stop gambling. On some level, she realized she was powerless over them, but she did not want to believe that. She kept telling herself, "I've had professional experience with this. If I can just find the right words to say to them, if I can just be the best possible daughter and sister, they will stop doing this." But over the years, try as she might, she could not find success with that strategy.

Adding to her distress and her shame, Belle found herself lending them money to cover their gambling debts on a regular basis. She loved her family dearly and did not want to see them hurting in any way. It did not seem to matter that her own life was suffering; it felt virtually impossible for Belle to say no to her mother and sister. The destructive pattern of their gambling and her enabling went on for many years, contributing to lowered bank accounts for all of them.

As time went on, Belle's physical health worsened, a direct result of the emotional and mental burdens she was carrying. She had gained a lot of weight and had begun experiencing severe headaches and stabbing pain in her stomach. She became depressed and lethargic, struggling with daily chronic pain. Even though her mother and sister could see that she was unwell, they continued their addictive behavior of gambling, expecting Belle to bail them out. And, for her part, she continued trying to "help" them.

One day, a work colleague told Belle she did not look well and asked if everything was all right. Responding to her friend's kindness just as a dry plant responds to being watered, Belle began sobbing, telling the woman about her mother and sister. She explained how guilty she felt about not being able to do more to help them. She also talked about her shame over being powerless to make them stop their gambling. Fortunately, Belle's colleague was able to give her a reality check regarding what she could and could not control. She compassionately suggested that Belle might want to talk to a counselor who worked with the families of people with addictive behaviors.

Belle did not want to think of her mother and sister as "addicts," so it took her a while to call the counselor her friend had suggested. But because nothing was changing, their dysfunctional situation continued and actually became worse. Not long after talking with her colleague, Belle was rushed to the hospital with severe stomach pain and, after a battery of tests, it was determined that she had a perforated ulcer and needed immediate surgery. Both her mother and sister came to see her the first day that she was admitted to the hospital, expressing their concern and sadness for her situation. However, although Belle was a patient there for nearly two weeks, they did not return for any subsequent visits. They did occasionally call her, but they were so busy at the casinos that they simply did not have time for her problems.

That was Belle's wake-up call. She realized during her lonely hospital stay that she needed to make changes in her life.

Back at home after her surgery, Belle's first baby step was to find the business card for the addictions therapist her friend had told her about. She soon began going to sessions on a regular basis. As she learned about her powerlessness over anyone other than herself, she became ready to let go of her own addictive behavior of enabling. She actually found it freeing to realize that rescuing her family had, in fact, not been helping anyone, including herself.

Little by little, Belle began to rebuild. She could see how small and constricted her life had become, and she examined new ways to revive her energy and excitement. Her list of things she enjoyed doing, although sparse at first, became more extensive as time went on. She identified her baby steps and began to enjoy taking them. Currently she is enrolled in two continuing education courses that are both nourishing her spirit and reawakening the enthusiasm she had thought was gone forever.

Liza and her mother continue to gamble regularly and are often worried about finances, but they are respecting Belle's firm boundaries by no longer asking her for money. As self-absorbed practicing addicts, they are only minimally aware of the changes Belle is making and are, as yet, unwilling to do the same in their own lives. Belle remains hopeful that if she can "be the change" she wants to see, she will eventually witness her mother and sister making some positive changes as well. For now, however, she is committed to the process of rebuilding her own life and to becoming happier and healthier, one day at a time.

Rebuilding Is an Ongoing Process

By now, you are beginning to understand the value of baby steps when it comes to rebuilding your life. These first steps generally correspond to thinking about something in a new way and investigating what you might like to try as new activities. The most important point about baby steps is that, in order to use them most effectively, you must meet yourself where you are *now* and not berate yourself for not being further along. When you can *say hello to what is*, rather than what you wish was occurring, you have a greater chance of being able to truly create the life you want.

There may be some activities you've been thinking about pursuing for a while and now feel ready to dive into. In that case, baby steps may not be needed. Trust your inner guidance and listen to the voice inside that tells you what you need to do. But if you're like many people who have experienced years of struggle as a result of loving an addict and are just beginning to put the shattered pieces of your life back together, you may feel that moving more slowly is a better fit for you.

Whatever pace you choose for yourself, try not to be in too much of a hurry for things in your life to change. If you've been stuck in some dysfunctional behavior patterns for a while, it might take some time to get yourself out of them. It is important to remember that rebuilding is a process that does not happen overnight for anyone. We are all works-in-progress, from the moment we're born until the moment we die—we are never really "done." When you can learn to enjoy the journey, without having too much attachment to the destination, your life will ultimately become richer, fuller, and more meaningful. Remember that rebuilding your life can be fun if you can be gentle and patient with yourself and take pleasure in both your large and small accomplishments.

CHAPTER 12

Survival Tip # 10: Don't Wait Until the Situation Is Really Bad— Reach Out for Help Now!

"If nothing ever changed, there would be no butterflies."

~ Anonymous

When people who love addicts of any kind finally reach out for help, they have usually been dealing with their difficult and painful circumstances for a long time. If you've been waiting to see whether things would get better without outside assistance, please consider getting help *now*, before they become even worse.

If this situation is just beginning for you, it is best to get some support as soon as possible so you don't make mistakes that could contribute to even more complex conditions. The earlier you reach out for help, the better it will be for everyone concerned.

Addiction in any form eventually creates nothing less than devastation in relationships, finances, health, and many other situations. Practicing addicts experience terrible life circumstances, the worst being the tremendous self-hatred they feel. On some level they know what they are doing to themselves and to those around them, and this knowledge contributes greatly to their lack of self-respect. A vicious cycle is then created: the more they do to contaminate their self-respect, the more they engage in their addictive behaviors; and the more they engage in their addictive behaviors, the less self-respect they have.

Having compassion and empathy for your addicted loved ones is not unhealthy. They truly are having a difficult time. What is critical to remember is that they do not have to continue living their lives this way. All addicts have a choice—they can continue to hide or they can reach out for help and recover.

The same holds true for you. As someone who loves an addict, your clear choice will be whether you seek out support now or wait for things to get worse.

How Bad Is "Really Bad"?

The 12-Step programs have a catch phrase to determine how bad things have to become before a decision is made to change: it is called *reaching a bottom.* There are several different levels of reaching a bottom. A *high bottom* occurs when addicts are still able to maintain their life tasks while continuing the dysfunctional behaviors. These people are able to go to work or school each day, and have not yet lost the ability to look after their basic self-care or participate in their interpersonal relationships. Even though they could probably continue the addiction for a little longer without experiencing major complications, they've become ready to stop their potentially damaging behaviors before their lives get totally out of hand.

A *low bottom* is reached when addicts lose a great deal in their lives such as jobs, homes, health, and family relationships, causing them to become desperate enough to make healthier choices. There are many points on the continuum between a high and low bottom, but because people's situations and personalities are different, there is no guarantee where the bottom will actually be for your particular loved one. It is each person's responsibility to know when they have had enough of the devastation addiction can bring, since this really cannot be determined by anyone except the addicts themselves.

Friends and family members of addicts also reach bottoms of their own. The one you arrive at will be similar to the addict's, though there will be some differences. Yours will start with the realization that, by not having strong enough boundaries, you have been enabling your loved ones to continue on their course of destruction. You will recognize that no amount of cajoling, allowing, persuading, or punishing has brought the change you want to see in them, and even more importantly, you will come to understand that your self-respect has suffered along the way. As you realize that the situation is not improving no matter what you try, you will likely become frustrated and angry, both with yourself and with the addict. You may also find yourself depressed and experiencing feelings of guilt, shame, and hopelessness. Please understand that whatever you are going through, your feelings are normal under these conditions. Self-awareness is the key: as soon as you perceive that you are floundering emotionally as a result of this situation, a better life can be yours.

This is your choice point—you can either continue to participate in the dysfunction for a while longer, creating an even lower bottom for yourself and enabling your loved one to continue the dangerous behaviors, or you can choose to come out of your fantasy that things will magically get better someday and understand you must take action to improve this state of affairs. Finding yourself some help will be a critical first step to choosing the healthier path.

Your Different Options

Although the numbers of friends and family members affected by addictive behaviors has risen substantially in recent years, the sad fact remains that it may not be as easy for you to locate support for yourself as it will be to find help for your addicted loved one.

Many options exist for people who are struggling with addiction, especially those with mind-altering addictions like alcohol and drug abuse. In most cities and smaller towns today, these addicts have the choice of outpatient counseling, detox centers, residential treatment programs and recovery homes, and of course a variety of 12-Step programs and other support groups dealing with many different types of addictive behaviors. Because this problem has become so severe and widespread in recent years, the field of addiction recovery has come a long way in providing a plethora of treatment alternatives for those caught up in the spiral of these damaging behaviors.

In fact, support groups are even available now for many mood-altering addictions as well. Some examples are Gamblers Anonymous, Overeaters Anonymous, Codependents Anonymous, and Debtors Anonymous, to name a few. For more information on any of these groups, or to see if any exist where you live, you can look them up online.

However, far fewer options are available for you as the loved one of an addict. As a result, many people with addicts in their lives are choosing the path of *self-help*. This path entails reading books like this one, watching related videos, and listening to pertinent audios that teach ways to implement appropriate lifestyle changes necessary to increasing healthy and holistic self-care. Other components of self-help can include receiving counseling from a therapist who is experienced in working with families and loved ones of addicts, or attending support groups such as the ones discussed below, which are geared toward people like you.

One choice is to attend meetings of a 12-Step group like Al-Anon, Nar-Anon, and Gam-Anon. You can also find support for your children in Ala-Tot and Ala-Teen. The format of these groups is similar to that of Alcoholics Anonymous and follows the same 12 Steps as other "anonymous" programs. Most of them have meetings you and your family can attend in person and others you can access online. For more information about these groups, go to http://alcoholism.about.com/od/alanon/Support Groups for Families.htm.

If you also grew up in a home with problem drinking and drug abuse, and are the adult child of an addicted, alcoholic, or otherwise dysfunctional parent, you may have been affected in a variety of ways known and perhaps unknown to you. To be able to talk with others like you who will understand the kinds of emotional scars that kind of childhood can cause, you might want to check out the 12-Step program Adult Children of Alcoholics (ACOA). For more information or to find a group in your area, go to http://alcoholism.about.com/od/adult/Adult Children of Alcoholics.htm.

The 16 Steps for Discovery and Empowerment is another option for the loved ones of addicts who want to deal with their own self-care. This set of Steps was developed by Charlotte Kasl, Ph.D. A recovering addict herself, she discovered she was having difficulty with some of the concepts in the 12 Steps, as well as the programs that use them. The 16-Step model can be successfully implemented both by people desiring recovery from any addictive behaviors and by those who love them, as it is based on spiritual principles germane to simply being human. To read the 16 Steps and to find a group you can attend, go to http://www.charlottekasl.com.

The professional addiction-recovery community is now beginning to comprehend the devastating ripple effects addictive behaviors of any kind can create in significant relationships. As a result, many residential addiction treatment centers have begun to offer shorter recovery programs for the families and other loved ones of the addicts participating in their facilities. These generally cover such topics as education about addiction, effects of codependency, the difference between helping and enabling, and appropriate and assertive boundary setting. Some treatment centers will offer these programs to people affected by addiction even if their loved ones are not currently attending their facility. The best way to find out more information is to look online for residential addiction treatment centers in your area and see what they include in their programs.

Another choice that is becoming more popular is to participate in outpatient counseling with an addictions therapist who is skilled in working with friends and families of addicts. It will be important for you to screen counselors and therapists to assess their level of expertise in the realm of family counseling. Some will provide a free fifteen-minute telephone consultation where you can discuss what is happening for you, ask any questions you have about how they might work with you and your family, and see if their approach is a good fit for you. To find a therapist in your area, or to locate one who will be able to provide telephone counseling for you, a good way to start is to type "addiction therapist [your city]" into a search engine and go from there. Most therapists today will have a website where you can get a sense of who they are, how they work, and what they charge for their services.

ADDICTION AFFECTS EVERYONE

We now know that addiction doesn't just affect the addict— and loved ones understand this better than anyone else. For every one addict (of any kind), there are upwards of 10-20 people who are negatively affected by the addict's addiction—these include mothers and fathers, sisters and brothers, spouses and partners, grandparents, cousins, friends, neighbours, colleagues, bosses, fellow students, teachers, doctors and even therapists, just to name a few. But aside from the addicts themselves, the people who are always the most devastated by the far-reaching and often horrific ramifications of addiction are the family members. No one is spared; everyone is touched by this brutal situation.

Although 12-Step and other support programs can be good points of entry when healing from addiction, what I've found in my many years of working with addiction in families is that most loved ones have already been down this path and, after a while, they end up feeling stuck in a cycle of spinning their wheels, trapped in belief systems that will never actually progress past the initial tormented realization of addiction. They believe that once an addict, always an addict—whether it's a drug addict, an alcoholic, a gamer, a sex addict, or even a people-pleasing codependent. They can't even imagine that the addictive behaviors can be arrested and that their lives can heal in any kind of meaningful way. In fact, by the time most people come to me, they've been living with addiction for some time and are still feeling confused, frustrated, exasperated—and stuck.

You don't have to accept that this is as good as it gets

What Do We Do Now?

What I hear from loved ones is, "We've tried so many different things. We've sent our addicts to rehab but they are still relapsing. We've gone to our own support meetings where we sit and talk about the problems we're having and listen to others basically sharing the same stories as ours—but there are no real solutions there. Nothing has worked and we're scared. We feel like we're at the end of our rope. Is there anything left to try? What do we do now?"

Loved ones share these helpless, hopeless feelings with me over and over again, especially as we begin our journey together. Perhaps you can relate as you're reading this. If so, you can see that you're not alone—there are families all over the world experiencing exactly what you are.

The whole family needs help to heal. Everyone involved needs to be able to understand the part they've played in keeping this treacherous dynamic going. They need help to be able to rediscover their resilience together, as well as their love for each other—which may have seemed to evaporate as the addiction progressed. At the same time that addicts need to go deeper into the reasons they've chosen to use addiction to medicate themselves from their lives, their loved ones also need to learn how to disengage from the roller coaster of chaos they've been riding right alongside the addict and start focusing on their own lives again. These new behaviors create the win-win solutions they have all so desperately been seeking.

You all have a role in your family becoming whole again.

Everyone Needs to Heal

This is precisely why I work with families as a whole, offering programs uniquely designed to help everyone in the family system—including the addict. It's important to look at it this way: if the addicts are the only ones to receive attention and help, but then they return home to the same dysfunctional family situation they left when they went into rehab, it's almost certain that one or more relapses will not be far away.

As loved ones, you need to understand is that you don't have a broken family needing to be fixed. Rather, you have a crucial role in healing your whole family— including the addict you love.

If you feel like your family is stuck in the quagmire of addiction and you would like to talk with me, go to the following link and fill out the questionnaire you'll find there, to give me some background about your family situation.

http://candaceplattor.com/intake-questionnaire/

In Conclusion

Let's face it—caring about someone who is struggling with addictive behaviors can be incredibly debilitating and difficult. The pain you've been feeling has no doubt begun to tear away at the very fiber of your life, creating problems and situations that you may feel reluctant to discuss with other people for fear of being judged and misunderstood. But the longer you maintain your private struggles and allow your secrets to keep you sick, the more difficult it will be for you to reach out for help. The first few times you try to call the number of a therapist or a friend, it may seem to you as if the phone weighs five hundred pounds, simply impossible to lift. But just like any other healthy life change, the more often you do it, the easier it will become.

If you are like most loved ones of addicts, suffering in silence has not served you well. Please remember that it is both self-caring and self-respecting to admit that the way you've been conducting your life isn't working well for you. Be willing to consider trying a different way. My hope is that by having read this book, you now have a deeper understanding of why you need to take better care of yourself, as well as guidelines to help you prepare to make positive and beneficial life changes.

Having once loved a person with addictive behaviors, I have found nothing as rewarding in my journey as saying goodbye to my own codependency and experiencing the increase of self-respect that liberation has brought. I deeply hope you will encounter the same in your own life as you continue to travel further along the path of self-awareness and transformation. As you practice holistic self-care and develop healthy boundaries in your relationships, you will feel increasingly free to allow your authentic self to shine through and to ultimately live your best life.

In Review

HOW TO RECOVER FROM ANY ADDICTIVE BEHAVIOR: ACCEPTING THE REALITIES OF LIFE

When it comes to recovery from addiction, here is the #1 question I get from the loved ones of people struggling with addictive behaviors:

> **"How can I make them go into rehab to get the treatment they need, so they never have to relapse again?"**

If you're the loved one of an addict, you may be desperately wanting to know the answer to this question—thinking that there must be *something* you can do to keep the addict in your life clean, sober, and safe.

The addict you love may be addicted to a *mind-altering* substance like alcohol and drugs, or struggling with a *mood-altering* addiction such as smoking, gambling, an eating disorder, Internet or gaming addiction, sex addiction, compulsive over-spending, or codependency and abuse in their relationships.

Sometimes it's a combination of several of the addictive behaviors listed above.

No matter how addiction is manifesting in the life of your loved one, now that you've read *Loving an Addict, Loving Yourself: The Top 10 Survival Tips for Loving Someone with an Addiction*, you're beginning to understand that life with a practicing addict is generally quite chaotic, even at the best of times, which probably don't happen very often.

But in order to decrease that chaos, we need to realize that we are powerless over the addicted person—as well as over everyone else, other than ourselves. It is that very *powerlessness*, combined with the *disappointment* of not being able to "make them change," that drives the loved ones of addicts to feel so bewildered and hopeless.

But by accepting the realities of life—such as powerlessness and disappointment—we can find the serenity we've been yearning for in our lives. By deeply understanding that the addicts we love are going to make their own decisions—regardless of how hard we may try to force them to do what we want them to do—we can come off that roller-coaster of chaos and start focusing on our own lives.

The wonderful ripple effect is that once we make the shift to accept the realities of our lives and stop pressuring our addicted loved ones, they almost always begin to make better, healthier choices for themselves too!

Remember: Accepting reality as it actually is will ultimately bring you the peace and serenity you've been wanting.

The Truth about People-Pleasing: Your Recovery from Codependency

The term codependency can mean different things to different people. Over the years, a number of authors have offered a variety of definitions for this difficult dynamic that seems to affect more people than we can imagine.

My definition is a very simple one: codependency occurs when we put other people's needs ahead of our own on a fairly consistent basis. In truth, when we are codependent, we are also people-pleasers who will go to virtually any lengths to avoid unpleasant conflict with others.

"I'm a Nice Person—Aren't I?"

Because codependents consistently put others' needs ahead of their own, they often believe that they are "nice" people.

But the truth may be that you are not really as "nice" as you would like to believe you are, because you are not saying yes to everyone else just to be kind to them. When you say yes (especially when you really want to say NO), you are actually protecting yourself from upsetting others by not making waves. You believe that this is the way to not have to deal with someone becoming angry or disappointed with you, for not agreeing to do what he or she wants you to do.

Although striving to be agreeable in all of your relationships could be seen as a self-caring intention, it is unfortunately not a healthy form of self-care when it is done out of resistance to unpleasantness.

We Teach Other People How to Treat Us

When you say yes consistently to another person, and when you accept any form of abuse as part of any of your relationships, you are essentially teaching the other people that it is all right for them to treat you that way. Although you might not be aware of it, you actually do have as much power and control as the other person does, because all of us can really only control ourselves.

It is only when you *choose* to give your power and control to another person that you begin to feel the sting of codependency, because the truth is that no one can disrespect you without your permission.

Your job is to treat yourself more respectfully; as you do that, you'll find that other people will automatically follow your lead.

Shifting into Healthy Assertiveness

If you are experiencing codependency and people-pleasing in any of your significant relationships, you have very likely been responding in a *passive* way when others have been acting *aggressively* toward you.

The healthy balance is one of *assertiveness*. This creates respectful, self-responsible communication without either person resorting to blaming, shaming or threatening the other in any way.

But change always has to start with oneself.

Aside from treating yourself more respectfully and saying no when you mean no, you will also need to become willing to learn how to deal with the negative reactions you might encounter as you choose to be more authentic with others. As you master this, you'll find that you no longer have to react from a place of fear in your relationships.

Remember: In order to become assertive, we need to be willing to tell other people the truth about how we really feel. It is also the most respectful gift you can give to yourself and to those you care about.

THE TOP 3 SECRETS TO STOP PEOPLE-PLEASING WITH YOUR ADDICTED LOVED ONES

Here are the **Top 3 Secrets** for stopping your codependency and people-pleasing while in a relationship with an addict.

Secret # 1: Stop being addicted to the addict's addiction and learn how to take care of yourself.

You'll know you're addicted to the addict's addiction by determining where you are on this simple gauge:

> *"When the addict in my life is doing okay, I'm doing okay.*
> *When the addict isn't doing okay, I'm not doing so well."*

When you're on this roller-coaster with an addict, the addiction takes first place in your life and in his or her life. The chaos of active addiction is ever-present for both of you—and you're aware that it's just a waiting game before that chaos either begins again or gets worse.

Remember: You need to be willing to come off the emotional roller-coaster that all addicts in active addiction are riding, and become ready to start looking after your own life.

Secret # 2: If nothing changes, nothing changes.

A while ago, there was a great commercial on TV that I want to tell you about.

Now, I'm not usually a fan of television commercials, but every once in a while there's one that really reflects something important in our society. This commercial, while seemingly all about cheese, is a perfect example of that societal reflection—maybe you've seen it.

The setting opens with an elderly couple, perhaps in their eighties, sitting at a dining room table. Their adult children—perhaps in their fifties—are sitting with them, waiting for their dinner to be served. The parents exchange a look of disdain between them, each rolling their eyes as if to say, "HOW do we get them out of here?"

The mother then gets up from her chair and slowly, with some difficulty, walks into the kitchen. We watch as she brings the food out to the table and ladles it onto her adult children's plates—a great example of enabling behavior. The "kids" dig in and enjoy their meal, seemingly without a care in the world, as they've probably done many times, for years and years … and years.

As we continue to observe this silly but awkward scenario, the narrator of the ad tells the parents—quite firmly—"Stop cooking with cheese!"

Whenever I relate this commercial to clients who are loved ones of addicts, they smile sheepishly because they can relate to the enabling that is going on in this fictional yet somewhat realistic family. They know that they themselves have been cooking with cheese for far too long.

Your job is to make it uncomfortable for the addict you love to remain in active addiction. This commercial tells us that if we keep doing the kinds of enabling behaviors that keep the addiction going, then the addiction is bound to continue.

Or—to put it another way—why should your addicted loved one ever wake up if you're going to keep hitting their snooze alarm?

Remember: Stop cooking with cheese!

Secret # 3: Stop trying to change another person and become willing to look at how you may be contributing to this situation.

Most people who love someone with an addiction feel very scared for them and, as a result, they want the addicts to change their lives as soon as possible.

If this is how you feel, then you've probably tried everything you can think of, including enabling them, yelling at them, and passively putting up with their often negative, manipulative behavior. You are also probably focusing all your energy on changing the addict and putting your own self-care on the back burner.

But because we live on a planet of free will, we are not able to control or change another person. *The only person YOU can change is YOU.* It is imperative for you to become aware of how you may be negatively contributing to the situation you've found yourself in—because that is the only thing you can actually change.

As Gandhi so wisely said, *"We must become the change we want to see in the world."*

Knowing this secret can help you understand the importance of looking at your own contributing behaviors, in order for you to truly affect change in your relationship with the addict you love.

Remember: Keeping these three secrets in mind and doing your best to implement them is what is required for you to experience lasting and positive changes in all of your relationships—especially with your addicted loved one.

Enabling an Addict is Never a Loving Act

It's important to remember that when loved ones enable an addict, they are often unwittingly meeting their own needs, rather than the needs of the addicted person.

People who are enablers are also generally people-pleasers who will go to great lengths to avoid dealing with conflict. Because addicts repeatedly become angry—and sometimes downright abusive—when they hear a "No" instead of the unconditional "Yes" they are hoping for, conflict can easily arise in these situations. When this happens, loved ones of addicts regularly give in and do whatever the addict is asking of them—even when they really don't want to or know in their hearts that it's a bad idea.

But the truth is that this is not what an addict needs. What the addicted person needs is to be given clear, assertive, healthy boundaries when their behavior is inappropriate in any way. What addicts truly need is for the people in their lives to love them enough to no longer support their unhealthy behaviors when choosing to remain in active addiction.

While it is understandable for loved ones to want to avoid the very conflict they fear—and often have no idea how to deal with in a healthy way—giving in to the addict helps them minimize their own anxiety. Although this may give them momentary relief, in the same way that addicts also get momentary relief when they indulge in their own addictive behaviors, succumbing does nothing to remedy the actual situation. As you now understand, *if nothing changes, nothing changes*—so when loved ones continue to rescue addicts by enabling them in order to ease their own apprehension, addicts generally continue to use their addictive behaviors as well.

This is never the best result for either the addict or the loved one.

You need to love your addict enough to stand strong, and to tell the truth as you see it. You will need to not only have clear boundaries, but also to let them know how their addiction is affecting you; the addicts need to hear it, and you need to say it in order to maintain your all-important self-respect.

Ultimately, the healthiest message to give an addict is that you love them so much that you are no longer willing to support them if they choose to stay in active addiction. You can let them know that when they are ready to choose recovery, you'll be happy to help them.

Remember: Enabling an addict really meets the loved one's needs—it is never helpful to the addict.

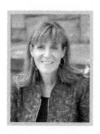

About the Author

Candace Plattor, M.A., Registered Clinical Counselor, is a therapist in private practice, specializing in addictive behaviors such as alcohol and drug misuse, eating disorders, smoking, gambling, Internet addiction, compulsive over-spending, and relationship addiction.

Candace offers individual, couple, and family counseling in her Vancouver, British Columbia office and by telephone worldwide. She also counsels family and friends whose loved ones are struggling with addiction, helping them to set appropriate boundaries and put more attention on their own lives.

Candace can be reached at 604.677.5876. You can e-mail her at candace@candaceplattor.com or visit her website at http://www.candaceplattor.com

Top 10 Survival Tips for Loving Someone with an Addiction

1. Come face-to-face with reality.

2. Discover how to love an addicted person—and stay healthy.

3. You cannot control or "fix" another person, so stop trying!

4. Stop blaming other people and become willing to look at yourself.

5. Learn the difference between *helping* and *enabling*.

6. Don't give in to manipulation.

7. Ask yourself the "Magic Question."

8. Know that "self-care" does not equal "selfish."

9. Rebuild your life.

10. Don't wait until the situation is really bad—reach out for help now!

CPSIA information can be obtained
at www.ICGtesting.com
Printed in the USA
BVHW080759040821
613443BV00005B/628